# Emergency Radiology

*A Manual of Diagnosis and Decisions*

# Emergency Radiology
## A Manual of Diagnosis and Decisions

Edited by **James T. Rhea, M.D.**
Assistant Professor of Radiology, Harvard Medical School; Associate Radiologist, Massachusetts General Hospital, Boston

**Eric vanSonnenberg, M.D.**
Associate Professor of Radiology and Medicine, University of California, San Diego, School of Medicine; Chief of Interventional Radiology, UCSD Medical Center, San Diego

Foreword by **Thomas J. Ruben, M.D.**
Associate Clinical Professor, Community and Family Medicine, University of California, San Diego, School of Medicine; Director, Emergency Department, Scripps Memorial Hospital, Encinitas; Course Director, Postgraduate Institute for Emergency and Primary Care Physicians, San Diego

*Little, Brown and Company*
*Boston/Toronto*

# Contents

# Foreword

It is a pleasure to so avidly recommend *Emergency Radiology*. I have coordinated courses for emergency room physicians for many years, and it is a common refrain to hear the uncertainties, apprehension, and frustrations of those of us having to interpret x-rays, but without formal training in radiology. This book is the answer.

The book is written for emergency (and primary care) physicians by those with extensive radiology training and experience. Even more appealing is that the authors have toiled as emergency room physicians themselves for various periods of time. One editor (J.T.R.) had formal training in surgery, and eventually headed the Radiology Section of the Emergency Room at the Massachusetts General Hospital. The second editor (E.V.), a board-certified internist and radiologist, functioned as a part-time emergency physician for many years. The authors have attempted to view films from the vantage point of the emergency or primary care physician; they have set out to fill the voids in training and to systematize our approach to radiographs. They have succeeded in grand fashion.

Much of the subject matter of this book is used in a highly successful radiology lecture series to emergency and primary care physicians in San Diego. These lectures are tailored specifically for the needs of emergency and primary care physicians; the overwhelming response by our course attendees has been for an extension of these presentations and for an organized presentation in book form. It is here, it is precisely what one would have ordered, and it fulfills a long overdue need.

*Thomas J. Ruben, M.D.*

# Preface

Clinicians, and especially emergency room physicians, occasionally must interpret x-rays in an emergency or ambulatory setting without the benefit of radiologic consultation. This is an unfortunate burden to the clinician and may have drawbacks for the patient. Despite the essential and frequently pivotal role of radiologic studies for diagnosis, the emphasis on radiologic training in the education of general physicians usually is insufficient. This leaves the clinician uncomfortable with many radiologic principles and findings; at times the clinician must act on his or her own radiologic interpretations, despite feeling ill-equipped to do so. In large part, this book is an outgrowth of the authors' own similar frustrations when working in emergency rooms prior to receiving formal radiology training.

The book is intended primarily for those physicians who lack the immediate services of a radiologist—the emergency room physician, the family practitioner and internist, housestaff in the wee morning hours—and for medical students, rather than for experienced, practicing radiologists or senior radiology residents. The book contains bread and butter radiology that is essential and practical for all physicians who interpret basic radiographs. Our intent is to provide a systematic approach to x-ray interpretation. This will help ensure that fundamental and often crucial findings and normal variants are not overlooked or misinterpreted.

The format of the book is structured to provide pertinent radiologic checklists and reminders for common (and sometimes subtle) clinical problems. When possible, the radiographic findings are presented as the patients present. The problems and radiographic findings patients bring to the clinical setting are highlighted; esoterica is avidly avoided.

It is intended that the transition from patient to film and back to patient will be a smooth one. For example, the ever-difficult evaluation of skull and cervical spine films should become more manageable with a systematic approach. Common but important dilemmas such as differentiating pneumothorax from skinfolds and fractures from normal variants are highlighted. Clues to the detection of cardiac versus pulmonary causes of dyspnea, and subtle findings of hemoperitoneum in trauma patients are points of emphasis. These and other important clinical points are highlighted.

The book stresses plain film radiography. In the emergency room setting, these are the films that are both requested and interpreted most frequently. The chapters on the skull, spine, extremities, pelvis, chest, abdomen, and thoracoabdominal trauma comprise the fundamentals of the book. A chapter on pediatrics, one on recognition and management of contrast reactions, and a chapter on radiography in suspected pregnancy address specific topics. A section on radiologic special procedures highlights the examinations that require specialized radiologists' and technologists' input. The major indications for these examinations are emphasized, rather than their interpretation.

We wish to thank Drs. Robert Novelline, Theresa McLoud, Linda Olson, Deborah Hall, and Alan Lurie for their assistance in obtaining radiographs. Our appreciation to Drs. Edward Webster and Folke Brahme for their contributions as well. Also our thanks go to Andrea Truax, Peggy Clark, and Debbie Lynn for their work in preparation of the book. Finally, the role and the tenacity of Little, Brown and Company and its editors—especially Chris Davis—deserve recognition as our partners in this endeavor.

*E. V.*
*J. T. R.*

# Contributing Authors

*Michael P. André, Ph.D.*  Assistant Professor of Radiology, University of California, San Diego, School of Medicine; Physicist, Radiology Department, Veterans Administration Medical Center, San Diego

*David C. Kushner, M.D.*  Associate Professor of Radiology, Harvard Medical School; Director, Pediatric Radiology Section, Massachusetts General Hospital, Boston

*Richard C. Pfister, M.D.*  Associate Professor of Radiology, Harvard Medical School; Chief, Section of Uroradiology, Massachusetts General Hospital, Boston

*James T. Rhea, M.D.*  Assistant Professor of Radiology, Harvard Medical School; Associate Radiologist, Massachusetts General Hospital, Boston

*Paul Stark, M.D.*  Professor of Radiology, Loma Linda University School of Medicine; Director of Division of Thoracic Radiology, Loma Linda University Medical Center, Loma Linda

*Eric vanSonnenberg, M.D.*  Associate Professor of Radiology and Medicine, University of California, San Diego, School of Medicine; Chief of Interventional Radiology, UCSD Medical Center, San Diego

# Emergency Radiology

*A Manual of Diagnosis and Decisions*

# 1 The Skull and Face

*James T. Rhea and Eric vanSonnenberg*

Trauma is the most frequent reason for obtaining skull films in the emergency room; however, the efficacy of these examinations has received much attention, especially with the availability of computed tomography (CT). In particular, finding a nondepressed skull fracture (75–80 percent of skull fractures) that has not extended to the skull base may be of dubious significance, because often there is no intracranial injury. Conversely, lack of a fracture on skull film does not necessarily correlate with presence or absence of intracranial injury. CT clearly contributes much more clinically important information about brain injury than skull films. However, availability and access to CT are not uniform. Many hospital emergency rooms still depend on skull films for trauma patients or CT time is limited (e.g., mobile scanners). The indications for obtaining skull films or CT developed by the Food and Drug Administration are seen in Table 1-1. Even using these criteria, there may be **significant intracranial trauma without a skull fracture,** or a **linear nondisplaced skull fracture may exist without intracranial injury.** It should be emphasized that if CT is available, it is more efficacious in suspected head injury, even if it means transporting the patient.

   **I. Method of interpreting skull films.** Since skull anatomy is complex, it is best to view the films in a methodical fashion rather than trying to "gestalt" them. Areas easily overlooked include:

     **A. Soft tissues**
       **1. A bright light** should be used.
       **2. Soft tissue swelling or** presence of a **foreign body** may help **pinpoint** the **site or sites of injury.** Occasionally, a superficial abnormality is visualized radiographically that was not clinically appreciated.

     **B. Base of the skull.** Check for
       **1.** Erosions
       **2.** Symmetry
       **3.** Demineralization
       **4.** Sinuses

**Table 1-1.** *Medical Indications for Plain Films and Computed Tomography (CT) of the Skull**

| Symptoms | Action |
|---|---|
| Low-risk group: Minimal initial signs and symptoms such as headache, dizziness, or scalp lacerations | Discharge to a reliable environment for observation—no need for skull images |
| Moderate-risk group: Initial signs such as vomiting, alcohol or drug intoxication, posttraumatic amnesia, or signs of a basilar or depressed fracture | Extended close observation; consideration of CT or plain films; consideration of neurologic consultation |
| High-risk group: Serious initial signs and symptoms such as depressed or decreasing levels of consciousness, focal neurologic signs, or penetrating injury | Emergency CT and/or neurologic consultation |

*FDA panel recommendations.
Source: Pamphlet outlining criteria for risk groups. FDA, Center for Diseases and Radiological Health, Division of Professional Practices (HFZ-250), Rockville, MD 20857.

**C. Facial bones**

1. Examine sinuses, zygomata, nose, and mandible individually.
2. Look for air-fluid levels in sinuses on upright or horizontal beam film.
3. Be sure to check for air-fluid level in the sphenoid sinus as an important and subtle indicator of basal skull fracture.
4. Check integrity of each bony margin.
5. Check for symmetry.

**II. Routine projections and normal anatomy**

**A. Routine projections** (Figs. 1-1 through 1-5). Several projections are necessary because (1) anatomy of the skull and face is complex, and different views reveal different structures to better advantage, and (2) fractures can be elusive and visible only on one view (Fig. 1-6). The battery of routine projections done on a patient varies from one emergency department to another and from one radiologist to another. A series of projections would routinely be selected from the following:

**1. Skull series**

a. Posteroanterior (PA) film
b. Stereoscopic lateral films of the affected side
c. Single lateral film of the opposite side (brow-up or upright to look for air-fluid levels in sinuses)
d. Caldwell's view (petrous bones and inferior orbital rim superimposed)
e. Towne's view (petrous bones above orbits)

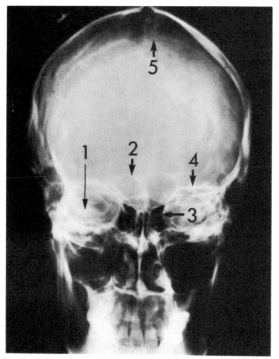

A

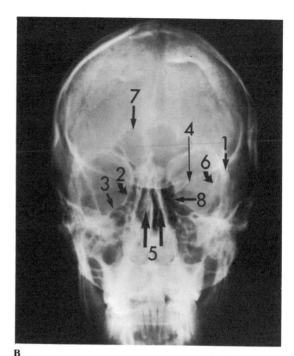

B

**Fig. 1-1.** *Important structures of the normal adult skull. **A.** PA projection (**petrous bones** project **through orbits**).*
*(1) Petrous bones. (2) Frontal sinuses. (3) Ethmoid sinuses.*
*(4) Superior orbital rim.*
*(5) Sagittal suture. **B.** Caldwell projection (petrous bones project at **inferior** orbital rim).*
*(1) Frontozygomatic suture.*
*(2) Lamina papyracea (paper plate) of ethmoids. (3) Posterior floor of orbit. (4) Superior orbital fissure. (5) Floor of sella. (6) Innominate line.*
*(7) Frontal sinuses. (8) Ethmoid sinuses. **C.** Lateral projection. (1) Inner and outer tables of cranial vault. (2) Vascular groove. (3) Lambdoid suture.*
*(4) Frontal sinuses. (5) Sphenoid sinus. (6) Sella. (7) Posterior margin of maxillary antrum. (8) Anterior margin of temporal fossa. (9) Orbital roof.*

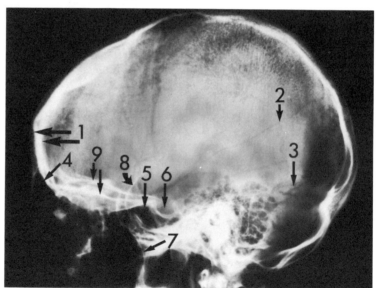

C

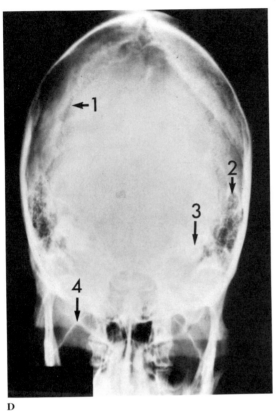

D

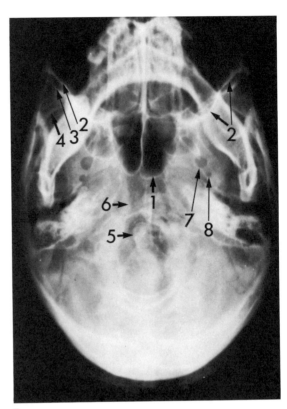

E

**Fig. 1-1.** ( *continued* )

**D.** *Towne's projection (petrous bones project* **above** *orbits). If the pineal is calcified, it will be seen optimally on this projection.* **(1)** *Lambdoid suture.* **(2)** *Mastoid air cells.* **(3)** *Petrous bones.* **(4)** *Posterolateral margin of maxillary antrum.* **E.** *Base projection (foramen magnum projects between petrous bones).* **(1)** *Sphenoid sinus.* **(2)** *Posterolateral margin of maxillary antrum, which is adjacent to No. 3 and No. 4 (dif-*

*ferentiation of posterior margin of orbit and maxillary sinus is by the characteristic sigmoid or S-shaped curve of the sinus versus the crescentic orbital margin).* **(3)** *Posterolateral margin of orbit.* **(4)** *Anterior wall of temporal fossa (smooth curve, convex anteriorly).* **(5)** *Odontoid process.* **(6)** *Soft tissues of nasopharynx and oropharynx.* **(7)** *Foramen ovale.* **(8)** *Foramen spinosum (carries middle meningeal artery).*

---

**Fig. 1-2.** *Important structures of the normal adult face.* **A.** *Lateral face.* **(1)** *Floor of anterior fossa.* **(2)** *Frontal sinuses.* **(3)** *Triangular zygomata.* **(4)** *Region of soft tissue adenoids.* **(5)** *Angle of mandible.* **B.** *"Jughandle" projection same as base view projection except lighter technique. Zygomatic arches seen to best advantage (arrows).* **C.** *Waters' projection*

*(petrous bones project at* **inferior** *margin maxillary antra).* **(1)** *Maxillary sinus.* **(2)** *Area of frontozygomatic sutures.* **(3)** *Zygomatic bones.* **(4)** *Lateral wall of maxillary antrum.* **(5)** *Inferior orbital rim.* **(6)** *Floor of orbit (* **same as roof of maxillary antrum** *).* **(7)** *Inferior orbital foramen.* **(8)** *Nasal bones.* **(9)** *Nasal septum.* **(10)** *Soft tissue over inferior or-*

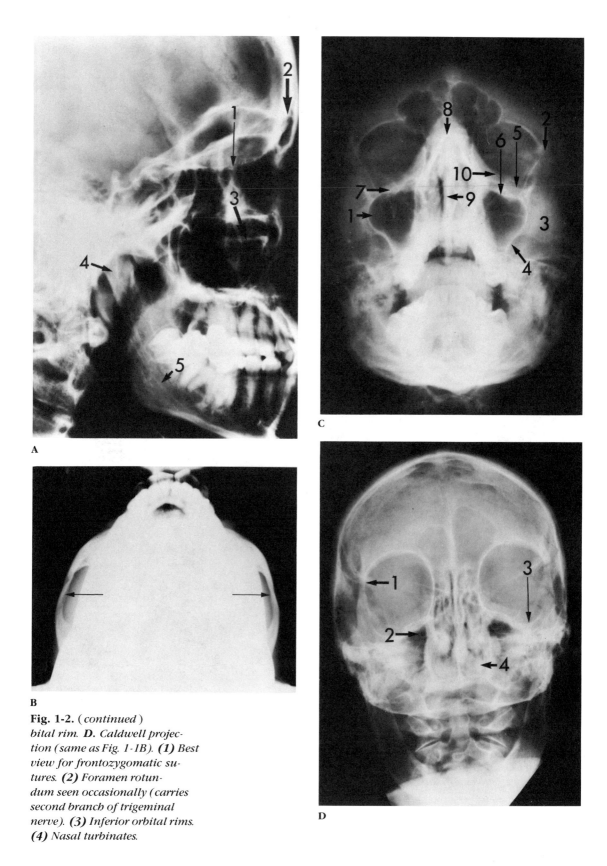

**A**

**B**

**C**

**Fig. 1-2.** *( continued )*
*bital rim.* **D.** *Caldwell projec-*
*tion (same as Fig. 1-1B).* *(1) Best*
*view for frontozygomatic su-*
*tures.* *(2) Foramen rotun-*
*dum seen occasionally ( carries*
*second branch of trigeminal*
*nerve).* *(3) Inferior orbital rims.*
*(4) Nasal turbinates.*

**D**

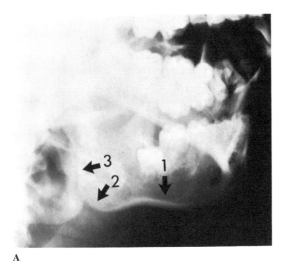

A

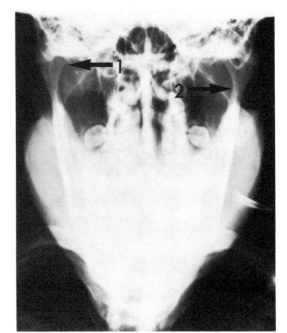

B

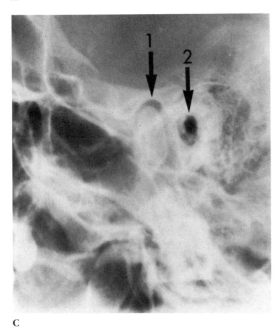

C

**Fig. 1-3.** *Normal mandible and temporomandibular joints.* **A.** *Oblique view shows the body* **(1)**, *angle* **(2)**, *and ramus* **(3)** *best.* **B.** *Towne's view shows the head* **(1)** *and neck* **(2)**. **C.** *Temporo-mandibular joint (TMJ) view with mouth closed shows head of mandible seated in temporal fossa* **(1)**. *External auditory canal is noted* **(2)**. **D.** *TMJ view with mouth open shows normal anterior motion of head of mandible* **(1)** *from temporal fossa* **(2)**.

D

**Fig. 1-4.** *Orbits. Lateral, Waters',
and Caldwell views, described
previously, are helpful (Figs. 1–
1B, C, 1-2A, C, D). Bilateral Rhese
views (optic foramen view)
shown.* **(1)** *Optic foramen.*
**(2)** *Floor of orbit seen best on
this view.*

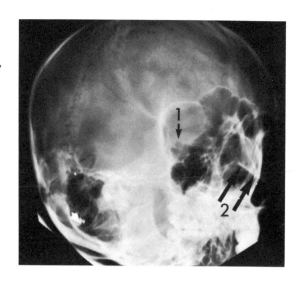

**Fig. 1-5.** *Nose. (Waters' view in
Fig. 1-2C to assess displacement
of nasal bones).* **A.** *Lateral view.*
**(1)** *Nasofrontal suture (**only
normal lucency perpendicu-
lar to axis of nasal bone**). **(2)***
*Nasomaxillary suture and neu-
rovascular grooves (these lucencies course almost parallel to
axis of the nasal bone; they are
not fractures. **(3)** Faintly seen
nondisplaced fracture at tip of
nasal bone. (Note: Lucency is almost perpendicular to axis of
nasal bone and therefore is a
fracture.)* **(4)** *Anterior maxillary spine.* **B.** *Occlusal view is
used for demonstrating **displacement** of fractured nasal
bones. Linear lucencies are sutures and neurovascular grooves
(arrows); this is not a good view
to visualize the fracture itself.*

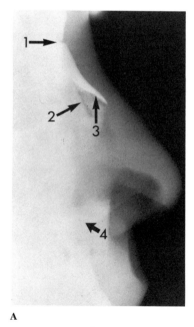

A

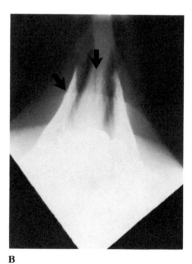

B

**1. The Skull and Face**

**Fig. 1-6.** *Linear fracture.* ***A.*** *A four-view skull series was initially obtained for this combative patient. The lateral and the two frontal views (not shown) did **not** show the fracture.* ***B.*** *The opposite lateral view shows the posterior parietal bone fracture (arrow).* ***C.*** *Since the fracture was seen on only one of the four views, an oblique view was obtained, which confirms the presence of the fracture (arrow) and illustrates some of the features of fracture listed in Table 1-2, page 31.*

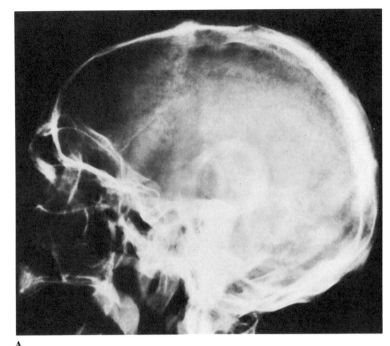

A

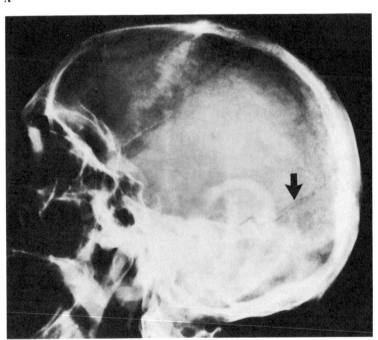

B

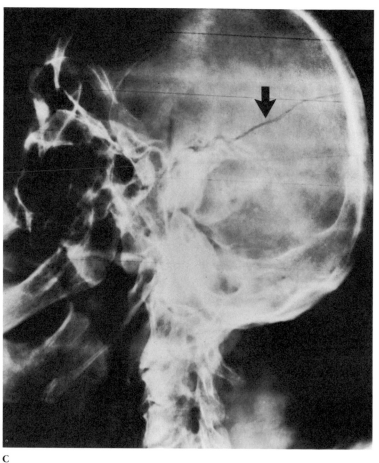

C

**f.** Base film (foramen magnum projects in center of
film)—**not included if there is suspicion of neck
injury**

2. **Facial projections** (see Figs. 1-2 and 1-3)

    **a. For survey of face, zygomata, and maxilla,** routine
projections include:

        **(1)** Lateral film

        **(2)** "Jughandle" view (base view with light technique)

        **(3)** Waters' view (petrous bones project at inferior
margin of maxillary antrum)

        **(4)** Towne's view

        **(5)** Caldwell's view

    **b. To survey the mandible,** routine projections include:

        **(1)** Lateral film

        **(2)** Oblique film

        **(3)** Towne's view

        **(4)** Temporomandibular joint views (optional)

        **(5)** Panorex film (optional)

**Fig. 1-7.** *Normal pineal and pineal shift.* ***(1)*** *Pineal.* ***(2)*** *Right outer table.* ***(3)*** *Left outer table.* ***(4)*** *Midline. Measure from* ***(2)*** *to* ***(3)*** *and divide by 2 to find the midline* ***(4)***. *The distance from the midline* ***(4)*** *to the pineal* ***(1)*** *represents the amount of shift. In this* ***abnormal*** *example, the pineal is shifted to the left by* ***more than 3 mm****.*

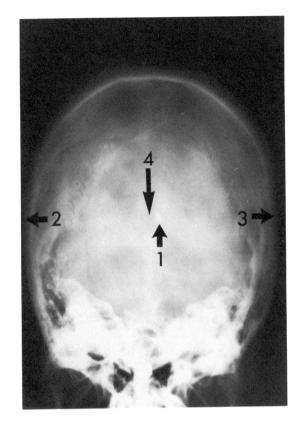

    c. **For survey of the orbits,** routine projections (see Fig. 1-4) include:

        (1) Lateral film

        (2) Waters' view

        (3) Caldwell's view

        (4) Bilateral Rhese films

    d. **For survey of the nose,** routine projections (Fig. 1-5) include:

        (1) Lateral film

        (2) Waters' view

        (3) Occlusal film

**III. Measurements.** Although there are many measurements for interpretation of plain skull films, two are particularly useful in the emergency setting.

    **A. Pineal shift** (Fig. 1-7)

        **1. Causes**

           **a.** Unilaterial subdural or other intracranial hemorrhage

           **b.** Tumor

           **c.** Prior intracranial surgery

        **2. Measurement method**

           **a.** Measure distance from midpoint of pineal calcification to outer table on Towne's or PA view.

    **b.** Determine midline by taking one-half the distance from one outer table to the opposite outer table through the plane of the pineal.

    **c.** Subtract measurement **(a)** from measurement **(b).** This difference represents the shift of the pineal from the midline.

**3. Significance of shift**

    **a.** A shift of **1 to 2 mm** toward either side is **within normal limits.**

    **b.** A shift of **2 to 3 mm** is considered **upper normal.** There is, however, overlap in this 2- to 3-mm range, and a patient with this much shift should be observed closely and viewed as abnormal if there are accompanying neurologic findings.

    **c.** A shift of **greater than 3 mm is abnormal** and implies the presence of a **space-occupying mass.** This finding must be interpreted further with such tests as CT, magnetic resonance imaging (MRI), arteriography, or radionuclide scan.

    **d.** Bilateral processes (e.g., **bilateral subdural hematoma**) may not shift the pineal because of balancing forces.

**4. Rotation of patient.** Slight rotation on the Towne's or PA view will not affect pineal measurements since the pineal is almost in the center of the calvarium. However, the patient should be positioned as accurately as possible.

**5. Is it the pineal?** The pineal position is such an important finding that there must be no doubt about its identification on the frontal view. If the pineal is seen only faintly on the lateral view, it will not be seen accurately on the frontal view. Innumerable faint densities can be construed on the frontal view from the normal mineralization pattern of the skull but should not be confused with the pineal.

**6. Where to measure within the pineal itself.** Measurements should be obtained from the midportion of the pineal calcification. This is particularly important when the pineal calcification is prominent.

**B. Sellar size** (Fig. 1-8)

**1. Causes of enlarged sella**

    **a.** Tumor

    **b.** Aneurysm

    **c.** "Empty sella syndrome"

**2. The normal volume of the sella is less than 1090 mm$^3$.**

**Fig. 1-8.** *Sella volume measurement. The Caldwell view usually demonstrates the floor of the sella in the frontal projection. Volume = ¹⁄₂ × A × B × C.*

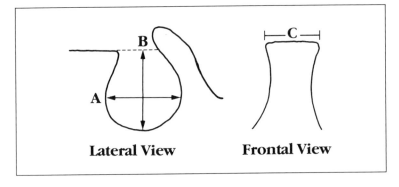

**Lateral View**  **Frontal View**

3. **How to measure the sella**
   a. Formula for sellar size = ¹⁄₂ × **height** × **length** × **width.**
   b. **Height** is measured on the **lateral view** and is the maximum vertical distance from the floor of the sella to a line connecting the anterior and posterior clinoids.
   c. **Length** is measured on the **lateral view** and is the longest horizontal line connecting the front and back of the sella.
   d. **Width** is measured on the Caldwell view, where the floor is seen projecting through the ethmoid sinuses. The floor of the sella is the same as the roof of the sphenoid sinus. The width is measured when the roof of the sphenoid sinus turns downward to form its lateral wall on either side.
   e. **Caveat.** The floor of the sella may be difficult to see on the frontal view. If there are no neurologic findings referable to this area and the sella is well seen on the lateral view and appears normal, no further action is indicated. If necessary, **tomography** may be performed to visualize the sella and obtain an accurate measurement. CT better defines the cause of any abnormality.
IV. **Normal anatomic variants and incidental findings that are frequently present**
   A. **Vault**
      1. Hyperostosis frontalis interna (Fig. 1-9)—localized sclerosis
      2. Parietal or occipital "thinning" (lack of mineralization) (Figs. 1-10 and 1-11)
      3. Variation in mineralization from homogeneous to coarse

**Fig. 1-9.** *A and B. Hyperostosis frontalis interna (arrows). This is a normal variation that occurs in 15 percent of women over the age of 40 years. The presence of hyperostosis in male patients should arouse suspicion of a pituitary eosinophilic adenoma or meningioma, since it is so rarely seen in normal males.*

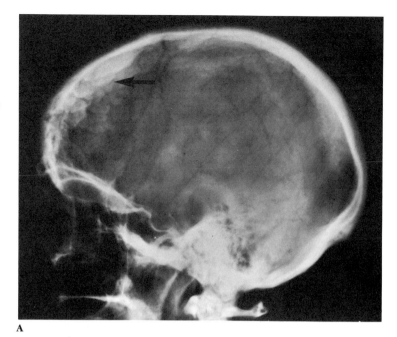

A

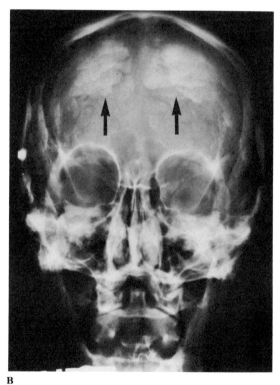

B

**Fig. 1-10.** *Thinning of the skull. This degree of lucency (thinning) can occur normally in the temporoparietal or occipital regions (arrow).*

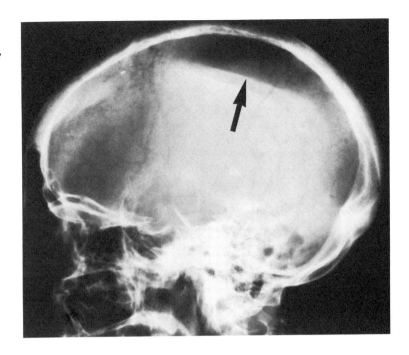

and variation in appearance of convolutional markings (Fig. 1-12)

4. Variation in number and visibility of vascular grooves (compare Figs. 1-9 and 1-12)
5. Asymmetry of venous (not arterial) grooves (Fig. 1-13)
6. Prominent inion (Fig. 1-14)
7. Venous lakes (Fig. 1-15)
8. Osteoma (Fig. 1-16)
9. Osteochondroma (Fig. 1-17)

**B. Benign intracranial calcifications**

1. Pineal (see Fig. 1-14)
2. Falx (see Fig. 1-15)
3. Habenula (Fig. 1-18)
4. Choroid plexus (see Fig. 1-11)
5. Dura (see Fig. 1-15)
6. Carotid artery (see Fig. 1-11)

**C. Sella**

1. "Bridging" of the sella (Fig. 1-19)
2. Sloping floor (see Fig. 1-17)
3. Sphenoid sinus pneumatization extending into dorsum of the sella (see Fig. 1-12)
4. Middle clinoids (Fig. 1-19)
5. Demineralization of the dorsum with age (Fig. 1-20)

**D. Sinuses**

1. Variation in pneumatization in adults (children and infants have proportionately less pneumatization)

**Fig. 1-11.** *Calcified choroid plexus and carotid artery, occipital thinning. The calcified choroid plexuses (1) are especially well seen because of the craniotomy defect in the skull. The calcified carotid siphon (S-shaped) (2) is seen well on the lateral view (A) and is also seen adjacent to the sella (3) on the frontal view (B). Also seen is occipital thinning (4). This lucency may also be seen as a normal variant in the parietal or temporal areas.*

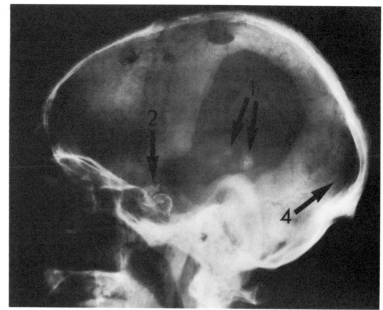

A

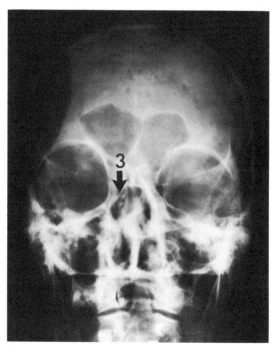

B

**Fig. 1-12.** *Coarse mineralization, convolutional markings. Mineralization of the vault is quite variable. The usual amount is illustrated in Fig. 1-1C.* **A.** *Example of coarse but normal mineralization.* **B.** *Convolutional markings may be quite prominent as a normal variation even in adults. Incidentally noted is partial pneumatization of the posterior clinoids (arrow).*

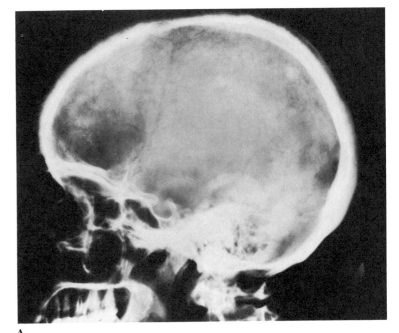

A

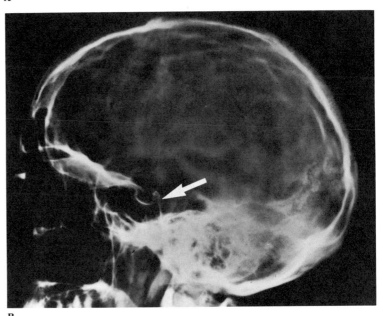

B

**Fig. 1-13.** *Asymmetry of venous grooves is a normal variation (arrow). Arterial grooves, however, should appear symmetric. Asymmetry of arterial grooves is an indication of meningioma. See Table 1-2 to differentiate between vascular grooves and a fracture.*

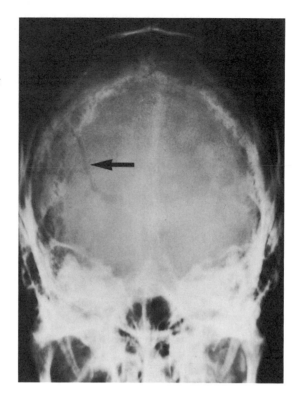

**Fig. 1-14.** *Prominent inion, calcified pineal. The inion (1), the prominence of the outer table at the confluence of the venous sinuses, can be quite apparent and hook-shaped or may not be seen at all. This area is the insertion of the ligamentum nuchae. The pineal is well seen (2).*

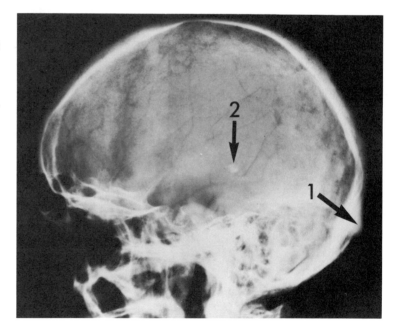

**1. The Skull and Face**

**Fig. 1-15.** *Venous lakes, dural plaques, and falx calcification. Venous lakes (1) usually are round or oval, occur in the upper one-third of the calvarium, and are joined to an adjacent vascular groove (2). Dural plaques (3) and falx calcification (4) are normal variations. A stereoscopic lateral view may be helpful to show the location of dural plaques adjacent to the inner table of the skull rather than within the brain substance. Practice in stereoscopic visualization is required. This view is optional.*

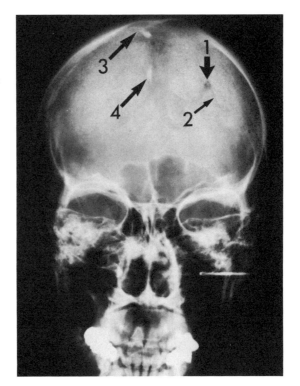

**Fig. 1-16.** *Osteoma. A, B. Osteoma of frontal bone (arrow). C. Frontal sinus osteoma in a different patient (arrow).*

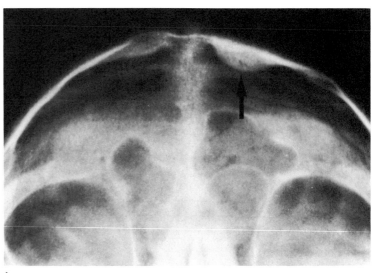

A

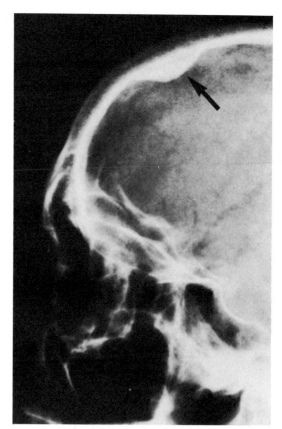

B

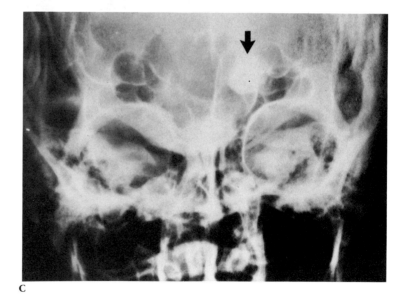

C

**Fig. 1-17.** *Osteochondroma of the lesser wing of the sphenoid causes asymmetry (1) in the frontal view (A) but is clearly seen as a well-defined "bump" (2) on the lateral view (B). The base of the skull is formed from cartilaginous rather than membranous bone, a prerequisite for osteochondroma. Incidentally noted is sclerosis about the coronal (3), lambdoid (4), and sagittal (5) sutures, another normal variation. Another incidental finding is the sialolithiasis, calcification in the left submandibular salivary gland, seen on the Caldwell view (6). The floor of the sella is seen well on the frontal view (7) and slopes slightly, a normal variation.*

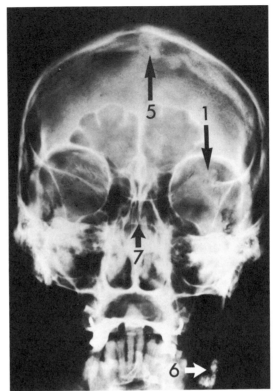

A

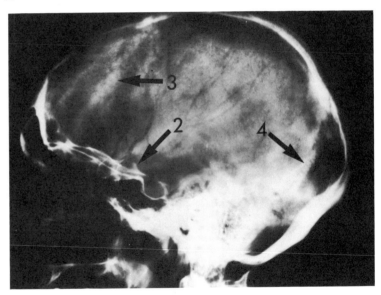

B

**Fig. 1-18.** *Habenular calcification. The habenula is the comma-shaped calcification (1) anterior to the pineal (2). It has the same significance as the pineal as a midline structure. Occasionally it may be difficult to differentiate between the two, which is not important since their clinical import is similar.*

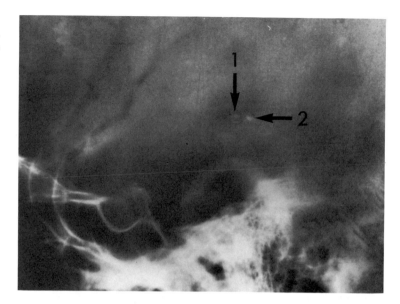

**Fig. 1-19.** *Calcification of the tentorium sella, middle clinoids. "Bridging (calcification) of the sella" may occur between the anterior and posterior clinoids or from the area of the middle clinoids as in this case (arrow). The middle clinoids may be seen as small "bumps" inferior to the anterior clinoids without bridging.*

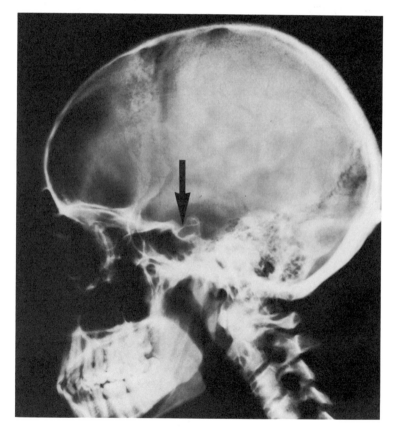

**1. The Skull and Face**

**Fig. 1-20.** *Adenoid tissue, naso-pharyngeal tumor.* **A.** *This 12-year-old patient has a normal amount of adenoid tissue in the posterior nasopharynx. Adenoid tissue can persist beyond adolescence and may be noticeable in the late twenties. In adults, this area is devoid of adenoid tissue and is smoothly concave (see Fig. 1-17B).* **B.** *This 69-year-old patient has a mass in the posterior nasopharynx* **(1)** *that looks like adenoid tissue. It is imperative to consider the patient's age if soft tissue is seen in the adenoid area. Incidentally noted is hyperostosis frontalis interna* **(2)**, *carotid artery calcification* **(3)**, *and "demineralization" of the dorsum sella* **(4)**. *Although the latter may be an insignificant finding in an elderly patient, it may also signify elevated intracranial pressure, which will be clinically evident.*

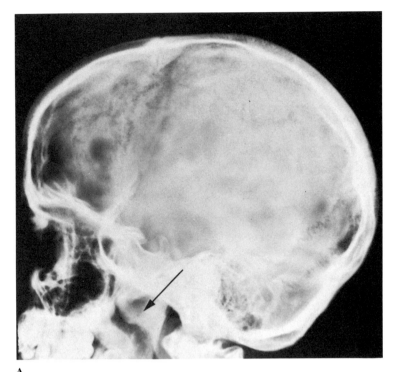

A

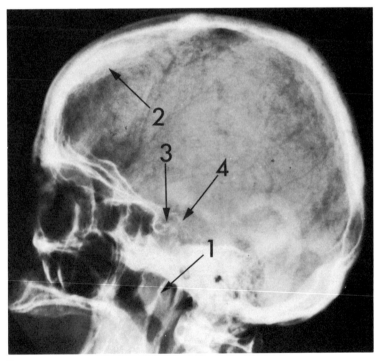

B

**Fig. 1-21.** *Mucous retention cyst. Characteristic findings include (1) the rounded density arising from the **inferior aspect** of the maxillary antrum with (2) **no evidence** of bone widening or destruction and that is (3) **convex upward** (arrow).*

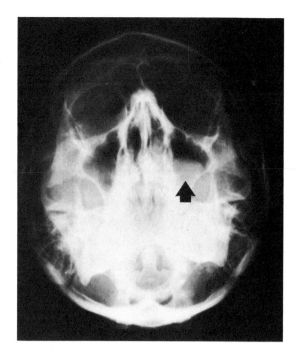

2. Mucous retention cyst (Fig. 1-21)
3. Osteoma (frontal sinus) (see Fig. 1-16)

**E. Petrous bones**

1. These are variably pneumatized (compare Figs. 1-22B and 1-23).
2. Internal auditory canals should be symmetric. Internal auditory meatuses should not vary by more than 2 mm in diameter (Fig. 1-24).

**F. Orbits.** Optic foramina should be less than 6.5 mm in diameter and should not vary by more than 2 mm in diameter (see Fig. 1-4).

**G. Sutures**

1. Metopic suture (Fig. 1-25)
2. Temporoparietal suture (Fig. 1-26)
3. Intraoccipital suture (Fig. 1-26)

**H. Soft tissues**

1. Pseudotumor of nasopharynx (Fig. 1-27)
2. Adenoid tissue (should not be seen after the late twenties) (see Fig. 1-20)
3. Soft tissues of scalp and neck superimposed over cranium (Figs. 1-28 and 1-29)
4. Matted hair appearing as swirls (see Fig. 1-25)

**V. Abnormalities of the skull and face.** Usually the clinical history and physical examination will give a good indication of the abnormality that will show up on the plain films. The patient may have experienced trauma, have had a seizure, have signs

**Fig. 1-22.** *Le Fort fractures.* **A.** *Le Fort, I, II, III. The drawing indicates the location of Le Fort fractures.* **(1)** = *Le Fort I,* **(2)** = *Le Fort II, and* **(3)** = *Le Fort III. The Le Fort classification represents a useful way to think about the weakest points that fracture in the facial bones. With a motor vehicle accident or massive facial trauma, however, an isolated classic Le Fort-type fracture is unusual. These fractures tend to be* **more complicated.** **B.** *The lateral view demonstrates fractures of the posterior walls of the maxillary antra* **(1).** *A clue to detecting this Le Fort I fracture is abnormal angulation of the hard palate* **(2)** *relative to the floor of the anterior fossa* **(3).** *Compare with the normal lateral view (Fig. 1-C), in which the hard palate and floor of the anterior fossa are almost parallel.*

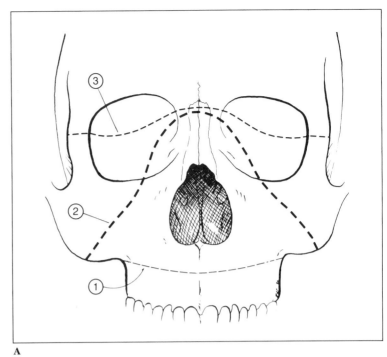

A

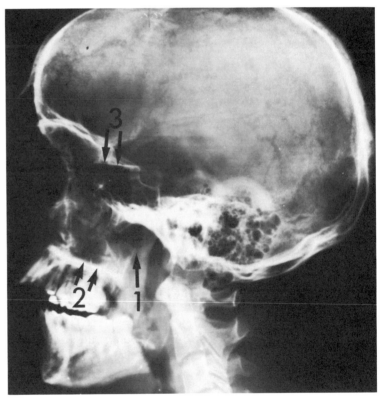

B

**Fig. 1-22** (*continued*). *C. In addition, there are zygomatic and orbital fractures on the right. The separation of the fronto-zygomatic suture* **(1)**, *the fracture of the inferior orbital rim (note asymmetry)* **(2)**, *and the fracture of the orbital floor* **(3)** *are evident on the frontal view. Also seen are two fractures of the mandible* **(4)**.

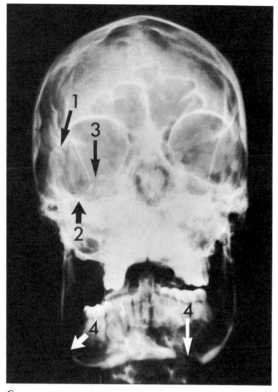

C

**Fig. 1-23.** *Glioblastoma of the temporal fossa. These punctate calcifications in the temporal lobe are in a glioblastoma. These calcifications are the only plain film findings of the tumor (arrow) and should be searched for carefully.*

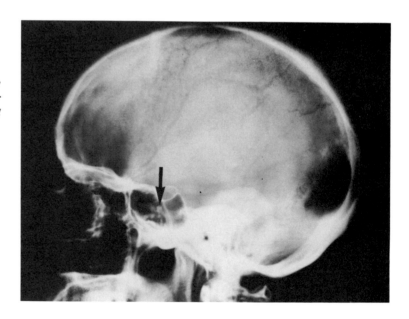

**Fig. 1-24.** *Acute sinusitis. An air-fluid level (solid arrow) is seen in the left frontal sinus. In the absence of trauma and bleeding and in the presence of symptoms and signs of sinusitis, this finding confirms the diagnosis of sinusitis. The internal auditory meatuses are well seen (open arrows). These are the usual sites of acoustic neuromas.*

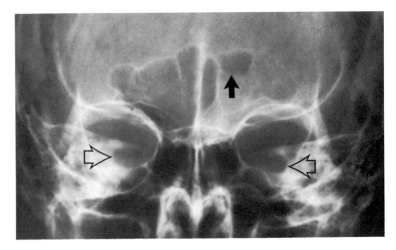

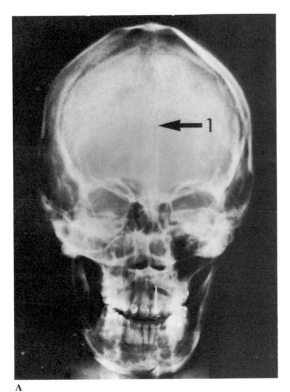

A

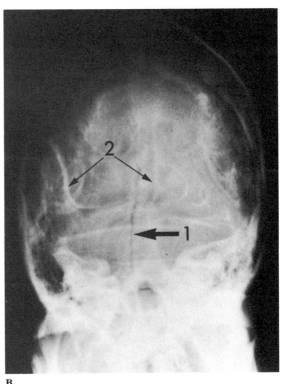

B

**Fig. 1-25.** *Metopic suture. The metopic suture (1) may be confused with a fracture. It is a persistent suture between the left and right halves of the frontal bone and has the typical radiographic appearance of a suture (see Table 1-2). Comparison of the posteroanterior (A) and Towne's (B) views leaves no doubt that this suture is **anteriorly located** since it **moves inferiorly with the facial structures** when the two views are compared. The swirling densities seen on the Towne's view (2) represent the patient's hair. This appearance is frequently seen if the hair is wet, matted with blood, or braided.*

26

**Fig. 1-26.** *Intraoccipital sutures, temporoparietal suture.* **A.** *This and other intraoccipital sutures, which are normally seen in children (1), may persist into adult life. The temporoparietal suture is rarely seen in adults on the lateral view. It is quite apparent in this child's rotated lateral view (2). These are generally **bilateral**, which may aid in differentiation from fracture.* **B.** *Incidentally noted is another finding in children, the incomplete fusion of the posterior arch of $C_1$ and $C_2$ (3) as seen on the Towne's view.*

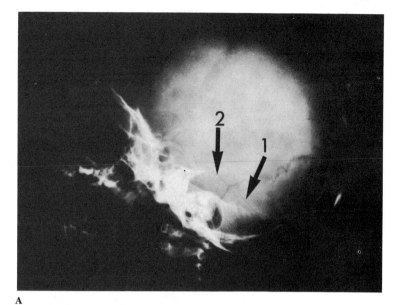

A

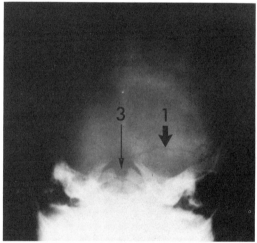

B

**1. The Skull and Face**          27

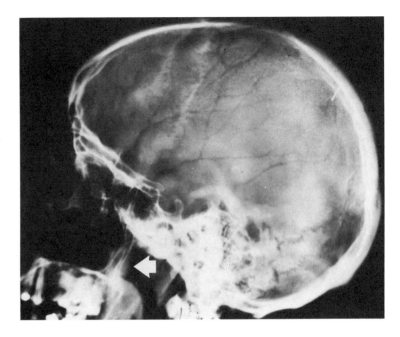

**Fig. 1-27.** *Pseudotumor of the nasopharynx. The rounded density in the nasopharynx is not a polyp or tumor. It is a superimposition of densities formed by the posterior aspect of the inferior nasal turbinate and the anterior and superior aspects of the coronoid process of the mandible (arrow).*

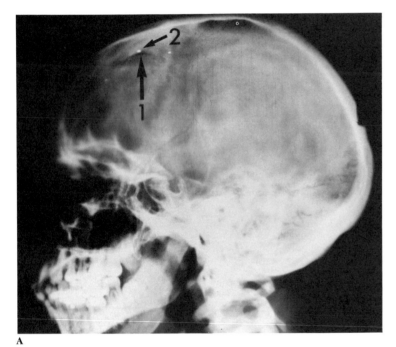

A

B

**Fig. 1-28.** *Scalp laceration may mimic a fracture.* **A.** *There is an abnormal lucency* **(1)** *as well as abnormal metallic densities* **(2)** *over the frontal bone. The lucency is not a fracture; rather it is air within a scalp laceration. The densities are foreign bodies within the scalp.* **B.** *A tangential view obtained at fluoroscopy may assist in defining such abnormalities.*

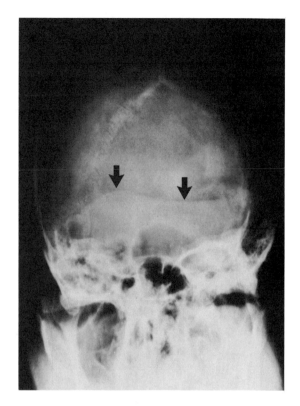

**Figure 1-29.** *Skin fold may mimic a fracture. This obese patient had a deep crease in the posterior soft tissues of the neck that became superimposed over the calvarium on the Towne's view and mimicked a fracture (arrows).*

of increased intracranial pressure or stroke, or complain of headaches.

**A. Skull trauma**

1. **Linear skull fractures** (Figs. 1-6 and 1-30). Linear non-depressed skull fractures may be confused with vascular grooves or sutures. Table 1-2 lists the features of each. **All straight lines must be viewed with suspicion.** Since the only "treatment" for a linear nondepressed fracture is observation of the patient for symptoms and signs of intracranial hemorrhage and increased intracranial pressure, it should be remembered that the crucial aspect is not the radiographic finding of linear nondepressed fracture, but rather the careful follow-up of the patient. Even if a fracture is not visualized, it is paramount that the patient be carefully observed and the family be instructed to watch for signs of neurologic deterioration after the patient is released from the hospital. With plain film finding or suspicion of intracranial injury, a CT scan should be obtained as soon as possible.

2. **Open fractures and basilar skull fractures** (Figs. 1-31 and 1-32). Like the clinical finding of hemotympanum, an air-fluid level in the sphenoid sinus on skull film implies a basilar skull fracture even if the fracture line is not visu-

**Fig. 1-30.** *Open skull fracture.*
*A. This linear fracture crosses the groove of the* **middle meningeal artery (1)**; *it greatly* **increases the chance of a subdural hematoma**. *The fracture extends to the frontal sinus (2).* **B.** *The upright Waters' view shows increased density in the frontal sinus (1). This implies that the fracture has extended into the frontal sinus and that cerebrospinal fluid or blood has entered the sinus. The patient must be treated with antibiotics as if this were an open fracture. The air-fluid levels in the maxillary antra (2) resulted from the blood or CSF entering the sinuses.*

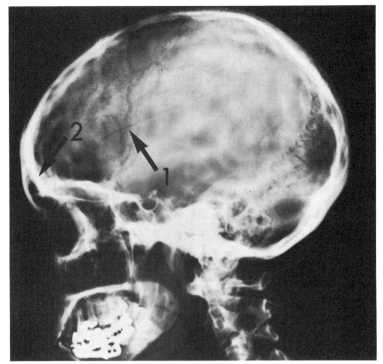

A

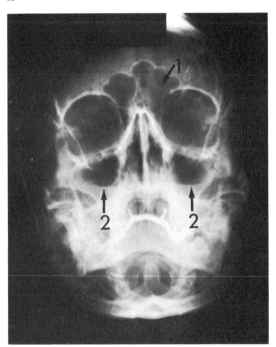

B

**Table 1-2.** *Differentiation of Linear Skull Fracture, Vascular Groove, and Suture*

| Criteria | Fracture | Vascular groove | Suture |
|---|---|---|---|
| Lucency | Most lucent (both tables involved) | Less lucent (only inner table involved) | Variable |
| Width | Thin | Wider and tapering | Variable |
| Edge | Well-defined, sharp | Smooth | Smooth |
| Bone immediately adjacent to lucency | No change in density | Faint increased density | Variable |
| Course | Angular or straight | Gently curving | Serrated |
| Branching | Less frequent | More frequent | Rare |
| Position | Anywhere | Characteristic positions (veins occasionally inconstant) | Characteristic positions |

**Fig. 1-31.** *Implied basilar skull fracture. This lateral view obtained with the brow up (a cross-table lateral film) shows an air-fluid level in the sphenoid sinus (arrows). Although no fractures were visualized, the air-fluid level suggests that a basilar skull fracture is present.* **The patient must be treated for an open skull fracture.**

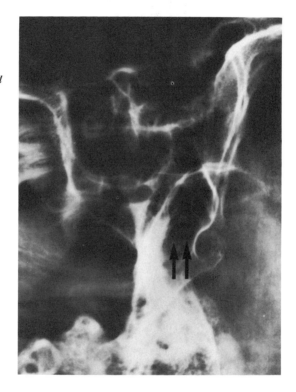

**Fig. 1-32.** *Depressed fractures. **A.** The anterior wall of the frontal sinus is fractured and depressed inward **(1)**. Because the inner wall of the frontal sinus is intact **(2)**, the patient did not have to be treated for an open fracture. Note the overlying soft-tissue swelling, a valuable sign highlighting the area of trauma. **B.** In another patient, the parietal bone is fractured and depressed (arrow). A tangential view should be obtained to assess the degree of depression.*

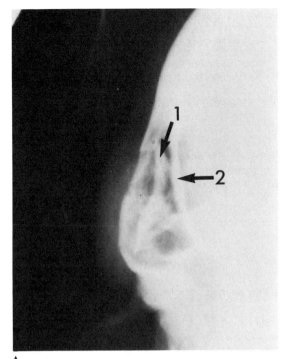

A

B

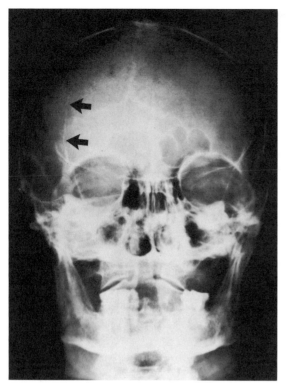
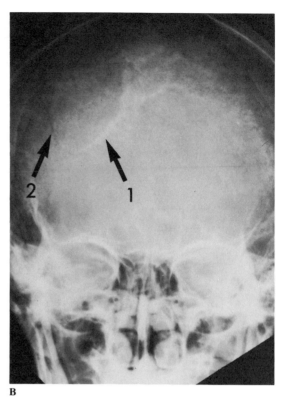

A

B

**Fig. 1-33.** *Depressed fractures.*
*A. The linear density was in*
*the exact area of the patient's*
*trauma and could be seen on*
*other frontal views. A minimally*
*depressed fracture is implied*
*(arrows). B. In another patient,*
*both the curvilinear density (1)*
*and lucency (2) of a depressed*
*fracture are seen.*

alized on the skull films. A patient is **treated for an open skull fracture** if an air-fluid level in the sphenoid sinus is seen in the trauma setting. If a skull fracture is seen to involve a sinus or if the patient has cerebrospinal fluid (CSF) otorrhea or rhinorrhea, an open skull fracture is implied.

3. **Depressed skull fractures** (Figs. 1-32 and 1-33). Depressed fractures appear different from nondepressed fractures. If a depressed fracture is suspected, a **tangential view of the depressed area** should be obtained because depression of greater than 5 mm necessitates surgical intervention to elevate the depressed fragment. Signs of **depressed fracture** include:

   a. **Overlapping** of fragments.

   b. A thin **dense line** caused by superimposition of the tables from the opposite sides of the fracture.

   c. Multiple fracture lines radiating from a central point (**stellate fracture**). Not all stellate fractures are depressed, however.

4. **Diastasis of suture** (Fig. 1-34)

   a. If a suture becomes separated, it will appear **wider** and **more lucent** than its mate or the other sutures.

**Fig. 1-34.** *Suture diastasis.* ***A.*** *(1) Diastatic lambdoid suture. (2) Linear fracture extending from the suture into the right parietal bone.* ***B.*** *Lateral view confirms abnormally wide and lucent lambdoid suture (arrow). The fracture is not definitely seen on the lateral projection.*

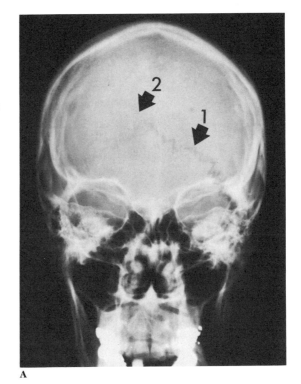

A

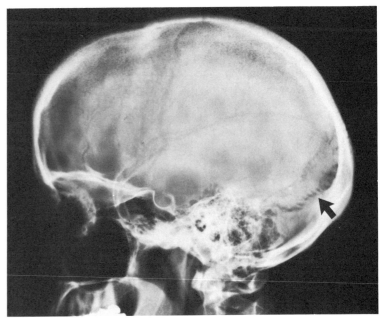

B

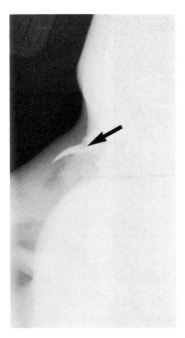

**Fig. 1-35.** *Nasal fracture. The fracture line, perpendicular to the axis of the nasal bone, is slightly depressed, as seen in this lateral view of the nose (arrow).*

**b. Caveat.** Slight **rotation** may cause an apparent discrepancy in suture width and lucency. If a suture appears diastatic, the finding must be confirmed on other views or by a repeat, correctly centered view.

5. **Intracranial hematoma** (see Fig. 1-7). Linear fractures signal the necessity of close observation of the patient for possible development of a subdural, subarachnoid, or epidural hematoma, especially if the fracture crosses a vascular groove. The only initial plain film finding suggesting hematoma will be **shift of the pineal** laterally on the frontal films. (**Bilateral hematomas** may balance each other and result in **no pineal shift.**)

**B. Facial trauma.** Facial fractures may involve the nasal bone, orbits, zygomata, maxilla, mandible, or any combination of these.

1. **Nasal fractures** (Figs. 1-5 and 1-35). The **Waters'** and **occlusal** views are obtained to determine **displacement** and adjacent injury, which may be difficult to determine clinically if there is significant swelling of the soft tissues.

   The **lateral view** is the best to determine the **presence or absence of a fracture.** Any line (lucency) perpendicular to the bridge of the nose is a fracture except for the posteriorly located nasofrontal suture. The nasomaxillary sutures and neurovascular grooves run along the long axis of the nose laterally and course obliquely and slightly more vertically than the plane of the bridge of the nose.

   The nasal spine of the maxilla is seen on the lateral view and should be checked for fracture.

2. **Orbital fracture** (Fig. 1-36). Orbital fractures may be isolated fractures involving the orbital rim, floor, or medial wall. The fractures may extend to involve the adjacent zygomatic, maxillary, or skull fractures.

   Repair of most orbital fractures is an elective procedure done following resolution of overlying edema. Even without a fracture, the edema may cause diplopia or simulate ocular muscle entrapment.

   **a. Caveat.** The superior and inferior optic foramina may appear to disrupt the orbital rims and should not be mistaken for fractures.

   **b.** Possible findings in orbital fractures include:

   (1) Orbital emphysema—implies fracture into either maxillary or ethmoid sinuses.

   (2) Stepoff may be seen in the rim.

   (3) Posterior floor of orbit not visible on Caldwell view.

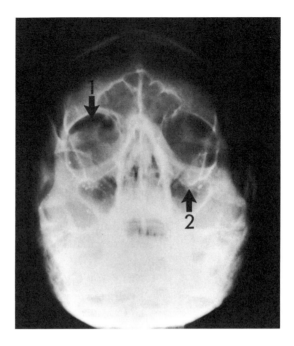

**Fig. 1-36.** *Orbital emphysema. On the right, orbital emphysema or air at the superior aspect of the orbit is evident (1). Although no fracture is seen, this finding implies a fracture into one of the adjacent sinuses. There has been an old orbital floor fracture (blowout fracture) on the left (2). The dots of increased density represent residual contrast from a previous myelogram.*

     **(4)** Anterior floor disrupted on the Waters' or Rhese view.

     **(5)** Bony fragments or soft tissue bulging into the superior part of the maxillary antrum on the Waters' view.

     **(6)** Asymmetry with the nontraumatized side should raise a high index of suspicion.

3. **Zygomatic fractures** (Figs. 1-37 and 1-38). Zygomatic fractures may be isolated to the zygomatic arch, may be seen as a "tripod" fracture, or may be involved with extensive maxillary fractures. Depression of the arch may compress the temporalis muscle and result in difficulty opening the mouth. A tripod fracture may be seen clinically as depression of the cheek.

    Findings of **zygomatic fractures** include:

  **a. Isolated arch fracture**

     **(1)** Best seen on jughandle view; may or may not be depressed.

     **(2)** Also seen on Towne's view, especially the posterior portion of the arch.

     **(3)** The suture between the zygoma and zygomatic process of the temporal bone should not be mistaken for a fracture. (The suture appears somewhat serrated, while the fracture will be linear.)

     **(4)** A depressed arch is asymmetric compared with the normal side on the Waters' view; it may appear as an asymmetric vertically oriented bony density on the injured side.

**Fig. 1-37.** *Isolated zygomatic arch fracture.* **A.** *The right arch is intact (1), while the left arch is depressed (2).* **B.** *Waters' view shows asymmetry of the zygomatic arches (1); the left arch is depressed. Note also an intact inferior orbital rim (2), the soft-tissue line over the orbital rim (3), and the roof of the maxillary antrum (4) (floor of the orbit) on the left. On the right, the infraorbital foramen (5) and mucosal thickening in the maxillary antrum (6) are seen.*

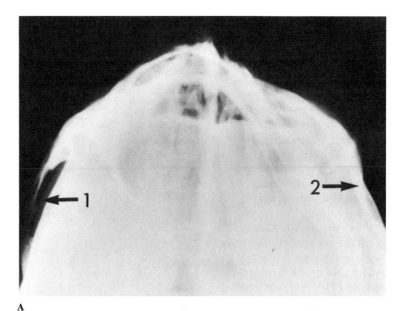

A

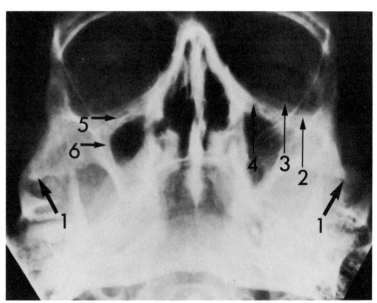

B

**Fig. 1-38.** *Tripod fracture. The components of a tripod fracture are* **fracture of the inferior orbital rim,** *fracture of* **zygomatic arch,** *and* **separation of the frontozygomatic suture.** *A fourth component is* **fracture of the lateral wall of the maxillary antrum.** *A. Fracture of the zygomatic arch (arrow). B. Separation of the frontozygomatic suture with medial displacement of the zygoma (arrow). Soft-tissue swelling increases the density over the right orbit. C. The acute angle represents a fracture of the lateral wall of the maxillary antrum (1). There is separation of the frontozygomatic suture (2) and asymmetry of the inferior orbital rims (3). Bleeding has resulted in air-fluid levels in both maxillary antra (4).*

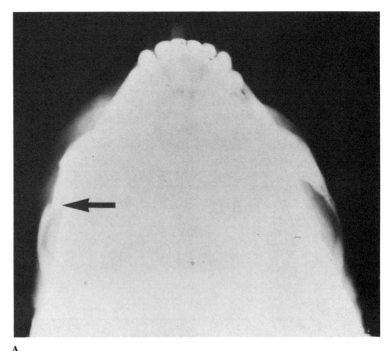

A

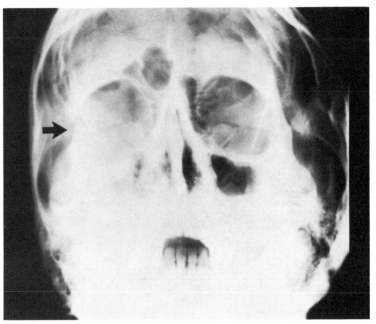

B

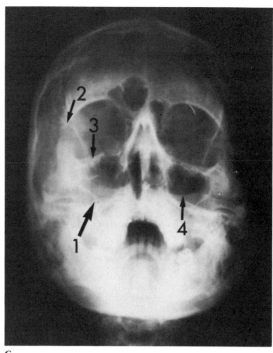

C

### b. Tripod fracture

    **(1)** The three components of this fracture are fracture of the arch, separation (widening) of the zygomaticofrontal suture (best seen on Waters' view), and fracture of the inferior orbital rim.

    **(2)** A fourth easily seen component is almost invariably present: fracture of the lateral wall of the maxillary antrum (seen on the Waters' view).

    **(3)** If the zygoma is depressed, rotation of the fractured zygoma may be apparent at the zygomaticofrontal suture or lateral wall of the antrum on the Waters' or Caldwell view. Either rotation or posterior displacement may be seen on the base view.

**4. Maxillary fractures** (see Fig. 1-22). The maxilla is most frequently involved when the other facial bones are also fractured. The Le Fort classification is useful for organizing these fractures, although combinations of these fractures are frequent. Findings with fractures of the maxilla include:

    **a.** Le Fort I—maxilla is mobile relative to the rest of the face on physical examination

        **(1)** Fracture of the lateral walls of the maxillary antra (Waters' views preferred).

        **(2)** Fracture of the posterior walls of the maxillary antra (lateral view).

(3) The normal virtually parallel relationship of the hard palate and floor of the anterior fossa of the skull is changed by rotation of the maxilla.

    **b.** Le Fort II—maxilla and nose are movable relative to the rest of the face on physical examination. Same findings as Le Fort I, plus a fracture is seen across both the nose and the inferior orbital rims.

    **c.** Le Fort III—entire face; maxilla, nose, and zygoma; are movable relative to the skull on physical examination. Fractures are seen across the nose involving the orbit variably, the zygomaticofrontal sutures, and the zygomatic arches.

  **5. Mandibular fractures** (see Fig. 1-22). If the mandible is fractured, it is most frequently fractured in two places; however, a single fracture may occur. Findings of mandibular fractures include the following:

    **a.** Fractures through the body or ramus are usually readily apparent.

    **b.** Fractures through the head may be difficult to see. The Towne's or lateral view should demonstrate asymmetry, and the fracture should be more apparent on the oblique views.

**C. Increased intracranial pressure**

  **1.** In children, suture diastasis is seen.

  **2.** In adults, there are generally no plain film findings, although an enlarged third ventricle may cause chronic pressure erosion of the posterior clinoids.

**D. Headaches, seizures, strokes, neurologic deficits** (see Fig. 1-23). Most frequently there are no plain film findings with these symptoms and signs. Occasionally there is a clue of underlying pathology, such as a tumor or infection. Depending on the signs and symptoms, further workup with other procedures will be needed.

  **1.** Abnormal mineralization (erosion or sclerosis) of the vault or floor

  **2.** Abnormal intracranial calcifications, which can be quite variable in appearance—punctate, stippled, or homogeneous

  **3.** Possible shift of the pineal laterally

**E. Sinusitis** (see Fig. 1-24). Membrane thickening may be seen as a result of either scarring or acute inflammation. The findings indicate the presence of acute or chronic sinusitis.

  **1. Membrane thickening. Caveat:** The lateral wall of the maxillary antrum slopes medially as it proceeds posteriorly. This adds some density along the lateral wall, which should not be confused with the more dense and more abruptly terminating membrane thickening.

**2.** Air-fluid level may be seen in the sinus.

**3.** Poor definition of the bony margins of the sinus and possible sclerosis of adjacent bone.

SELECTED READINGS

Baker SR, Gaylord GM, Lantos G, et al. Emergency skull radiography: Effect of restrictive criteria on skull radiography and CT use. Radiology 156: 409, 1985.

Cohen RA, Kaufman RA, Myers PA, et al. Cranial computed tomography in the abused child with head injury. AJNR 6:883, 1985.

Garniak A, Feivel M, Hertz M, et al. Skull x-rays in head trauma: Are they still necessary? A review of 1000 cases. Eur J Radiol 6:89, 1986.

Hryshko FG, Deeb ZL. Computed tomography in acute head injuries. Radiology 152:556, 1984.

Terrier F, Raveh J, Burckhardt B. Conventional tomography and computed tomography for the diagnosis of fronto-basal fractures. Radiology 154: 566, 1985.

Thornbury JR, Campbell JA, Masters SJ, et al. Skull fracture and the low risk of intracranial sequelae in minor head trauma. AJNR 5:459, 1984.

Toutant SM, Klauber MR, Marshall LF, et al. Absent or compressed basal cisterns on first CT scan: Ominous predictors of outcome in severe head injury. Radiology 155:858, 1985.

Tsai FY, Teal JS, Hieshima GB. *Neuroradiology of Head Trauma.* Baltimore: University Park Press, 1983. P. 416.

van Dongen KJ, Braakman R, Gelpke GJ. Prognostic value of computerized tomography in comatose head-injured patients. Radiology 152:854, 1984.

Zimmerman RA, Bilaniuk LT, Hackney DB, et al. Head injury: Early results of comparing CT and high-field MR. AJNR 7:757, 1986.

# 2    The Cervical Spine

*James T. Rhea and Eric vanSonnenberg*

Catastrophic results may be avoided by correct and expeditious interpretation of cervical spine radiographs. Meticulous filming and accurate diagnosis are paramount in all suspected cervical spine injuries. When an unstable injury has occurred, the spinal cord may be damaged if the trauma and its extent are not appreciated. In the severely injured patient, a portable lateral examination of the cervical spine should be obtained initially. A complete five-view examination is indicated when injury is suspected, since subtle findings may not be seen on any single view. Unstable injuries may occur even in ambulatory patients. Use of a cervical collar and care in moving the patient offer a degree of protection. With a patient who has a suspected injury, the cervical spine should be protected until there is reasonable radiographic certainty that no major injury has occurred.

### I. Indications for cervical spine examination
    **A.** Neurologic signs
    **B.** Pain, which may be caused by
        **1.** Trauma
        **2.** Degenerative changes
        **3.** Muscle spasm
        **4.** Tumor
### II. Routine views (Fig. 2-1)
    **A. Adult.** Anteroposterior (AP), lateral, both obliques, and AP open-mouth or odontoid views.
    **B. Pediatric.** AP and lateral views.
    **C. Caveat.** Especially following trauma, it is important to visualize **all seven** vertebrae in the lateral view to exclude fracture or dislocation at C7. In the face of trauma and lower cervical spine pain or neurologic signs, no patient should be sent home without a complete examination of the C7–T1 level.
### III. Clues to normal appearance
    **A.** All seven cervical vertebrae must be seen.
    **B.** On the lateral view, there should be a normal lordosis.
    **C.** The respective anterior and posterior margins of the vertebral bodies should align and form smooth curves on the lateral view.

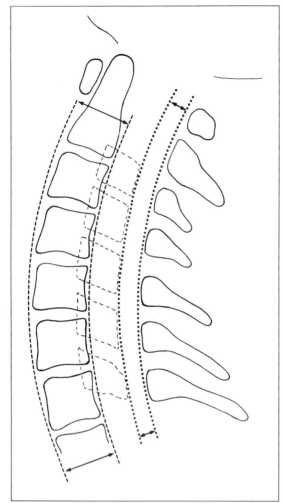

**A**

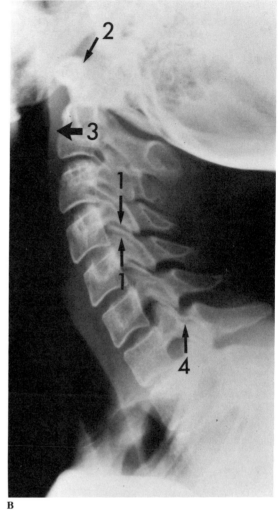

**B**

**Fig. 2-1.** *Normal cervical spine. The following checklist of normal findings should be an integral part of analyzing all cervical spine series.* **A. *Normal curves of alignment (dotted lines).*** *Anterior and posterior margins of vertebral bodies, posterior margins of articular pillars from C2 through C6, and posterior margin of spinal canal should align as smooth curves.* **B. *Normal lateral view.*** *Paired facet joints will either superimpose and appear as a single lucent line or appear as paired lucent lines that are parallel, with one immediately superior to the other (1). Slight rotation will result in one facet*

*joint appearing correspondingly anterior to the other. In a true lateral view, the neural foramina are not seen. The distance between the spinous processes varies from level to level, but the amount of variation is slight. The distance between the odontoid and the anterior arch of C1 is 3mm or less in adults and 5 mm or less in infants and children (2). The retropharyngeal soft tissues above the level of the vocal cords should not exceed 4 mm in thickness in adults (3). A thickness greater than 4 mm is a sensitive index of abnormality (e.g., edema, pus, hemorrhage). In children this distance is variable and depends on the degree*

*of flexion of the head and the phase of respiration. Below the level of the vocal cords, the thickness of the soft tissues is quite variable and depends on the patient's age and the position of the neck (see Fig. 2-12). Adenoid tissues are prominent in children and adolescents but should not be visible beyond the late twenties (not seen in this view, see Fig. 2-22). A notch is seen in the superior facet of C7, a normal finding not to be confused with fracture (4).* **C. *Normal anteroposterior (AP) view.*** *The pedicles (1) and spinous processes (2) should align in a straight line or smooth curve. Bifid spinous processes*

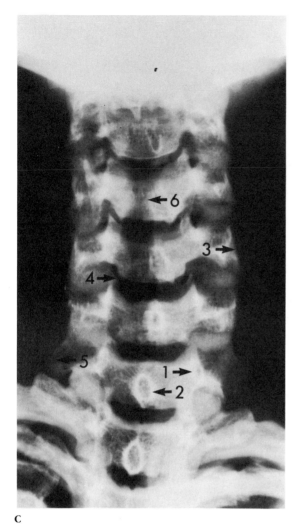

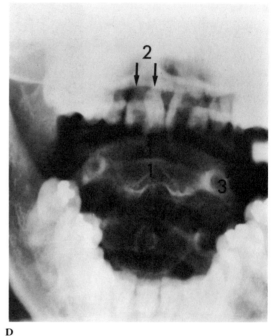

**C**

*may appear to disrupt this line;
these are common normal variants. The articular pillars are
not seen individually; rather,
they overlap to form a smooth
undulating lateral border (3).
The "joints of Luschka" are seen
well in the AP view (4); the
transverse processes may be seen
laterally in the upper cervical
spine; C7 is the largest transverse
process. The transverse processes
in the cervical spine slope inferiorly (5); those in the thoracic spine slope superiorly to
articulate with the angle of the
ribs (see Fig. 2-3). This difference
helps distinguish cervical from
thoracic vertebrae. The lucency
of the tracheal air column is*

**D**

*superimposed and should be
checked for position and symmetry, especially at the level of
the vocal chords (6). This air
column should not be mistaken
for a fracture.* **D. Odontoid
view (AP).** *The AP view (2C)
does not demonstrate the odontoid because of the overlying
mandible. The open-mouth view
best demonstrates the odontoid
in the AP projection. The odontoid is best seen when the teeth
(1) and occiput (2) superimpose. Positioning is difficult;
frequently, the teeth and occiput
are not exactly superimposed.
The normal odontoid has no
transverse lucency or abrupt tilt.
If there is no rotation or scolio-*

*sis, the lateral aspect of the ar-
ticular facets of C1 and C2 align
exactly on each other (3).* **E.
Oblique views (only one is
shown).** *In this view, the left
laminae (1), the left neural foramina (2), and the right pedicles (3) align in smooth curves.
The spinous processes may or
may not be seen, depending on
the degree of rotation. They are
well seen to the left in this view
(4). The left articular pillars
(5) are superimposed over the
left laminae, and the left facet
joints are seen in their normal
alignment (6). The right facet
joints are superimposed as linear lucencies over the vertebral
bodies (7). The right transverse*

**Fig. 2-1.** (*continued*) *processes (best seen with the bright light) project to the right of the vertebral body (8). The superimposed left pedicles and right laminae form the upper and lower borders of the neural foramina.*

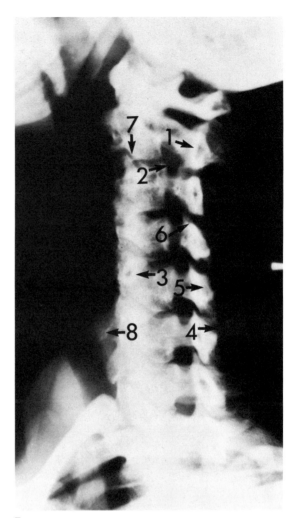

E

D. The distance between spinous processes should be relatively even; widening at a particular site suggests damage (although widening may also be a developmental variation).

E. On the AP view, the spinous processes should align vertically one under the other; malalignment is a clue to an underlying abnormality.

IV. Special views (Table 2-1)

A. Swimmer's view (Fig. 2-2) demonstrates C7–T1.

B. **Repeat lateral** view (if the initial view was unsatisfactory) while pulling down on the patient's arms permits visualization of C7–T1.

C. Pillar view (Fig. 2-3) shows the articular pillar en face and to best advantage.

D. Flexion and extension views (Fig. 2-4)

1. **Indication.** Obtain when routine examination or

**Fig. 2-2.** *Normal swimmer's view. The patient is positioned as if swimming with one arm extended above the head and the other by the side. T1 is identified by its association with the first rib. In this patient, the first rib overlies the upper portion of the T1 vertebral body (1), and the clavicle overlies the C6–C7 disc space (2). The normal alignment of the vertebral bodies, articular pillars, and facet joints is seen.*

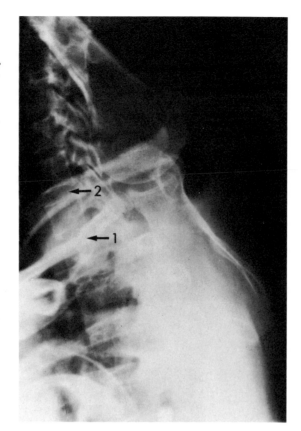

**Table 2-1.** *Indications for Special Views of the Cervical Spine*

| Clinical or radiographic question | Special views |
|---|---|
| Inability to visualize C7 | Swimmer's view, repeat lateral, with arm pull, tomography, or computed tomography (CT) |
| Rule out fracture of articular pillar | Pillar view, tomography, or CT |
| Rule out ligamentous instability | Flexion and extension views |
| What is extent of lesion? | Tomography or CT |
| Is there fracture in the axial plane? | Tomography |
| Are there fracture fragments near the cord? | CT |

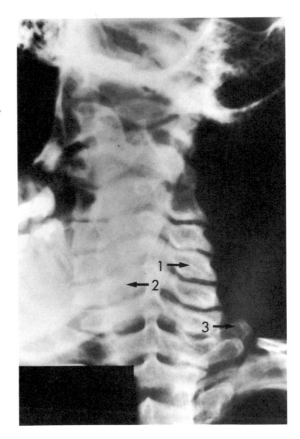

**Fig. 2-3.** *Pillar view. The patient is supine with the head turned first to one side and then to the other to remove the superimposed mandible. The x-ray tube is angled to parallel the facet joints and the two films are obtained. In this patient, the head is turned toward the right, and the mandible overlies the right articular pillars. In addition to the articular pillars (1), the laminae (2) are well seen. (The left laminae are foreshortened because of rotation.) The vertebral bodies are projected obliquely and are obscured. The articular pillars of C1 and C2 are not well seen. The lateral margin of the articular pillars normally varies in shape. T1 is easily identified because of its superiorly directed transverse processes (3).*

clinical findings raise the question of ligamentous injury.

**2. Abnormal findings**

    **a.** Subluxation of one vertebral body on another

    **b.** Disproportionate widening of distance between two spinous processes or two laminae

    **c.** Widening of a facet joint

**3. Caveat.** The patient should gently and voluntarily flex and extend to prevent injury to the cord. The patient who is unable to flex or extend voluntarily should be manipulated under fluoroscopic control only and with supervision of the clinician.

**E.** Tomography or computed tomography (CT)—indications

    **1.** Uncertainty of a fracture on routine views

    **2.** Determination of the extent of a fracture

    **3.** Determination of position of fracture fragments

    **4.** Visualization of the lower cervical spine if other methods fail

**V. Normal variants and incidental findings,** which should not be confused with significant abnormalities

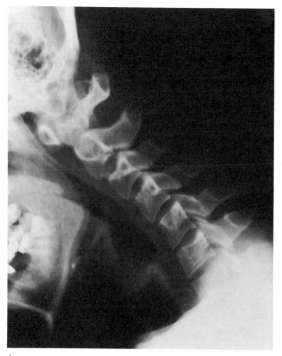

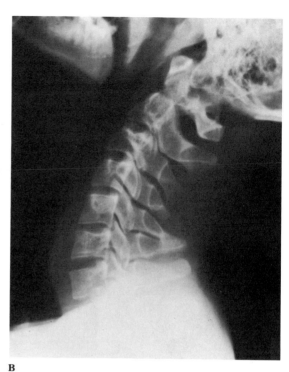

A

B

**Fig. 2-4.** *Flexion **(A)** and normal extension **(B)** views. The distance between the spinous processes varies minimally at different levels. In flexion, the C2 vertebral body may move anterior to C3 slightly. The same finding may be seen at C3–C4 and C4–C5. This normal variation, called pseudosubluxation, is accentuated in younger patients because of normal ligamentous laxity (see Fig. 2-12). Note the **smooth** curve of the posterior margin of the spinal canal and that the anterior arch of C1 is closely applied to the odontoid.*

**Fig. 2-5.** *Aplasia of the lateral portion of the C1 arch. Aplasia of the lateral aspects of the C1 ring is a normal variant (arrow). In this case only the anterior arch and spinous process have ossified. This is not a fracture.*

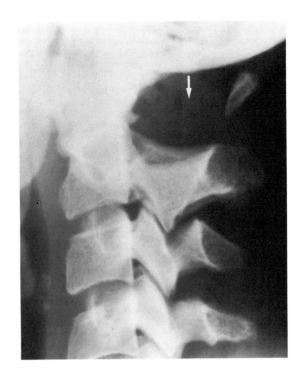

A. Vertebrae

1. **Aplasia** of part of a posterior arch (Figs. 2-5 and 2-6).

2. **Secondary ossicles** above or below the anterior arch of C1 (Fig. 2-7).

3. **Unfused apophyses** at anterior margins of vertebral bodies, facets, and spinous or transverse processes (Fig. 2-8).

4. **Displacement** of a lateral mass of C1 relative to facet of C2 may be normal. It has a characteristic appearance, and should not be confused with a Jefferson fracture (Figs. 2-9, 2-10, and 2-11).

5. **Pseudosubluxation** (anterior subluxation usually of C2 on C3) reflects normal ligamentous laxity in **children** (Fig. 2-12). If symptoms suggest ligamentous injury, flexion and extension views should be obtained.

6. **Backward tilt of the odontoid** (see Fig. 2-8) is a normal variant but should prompt a careful search for a fracture at the base of the odontoid.

7. **Congenital fusion** of vertebral bodies with or without fusion of articular pillars and posterior arch may occur (Fig. 2-13).

8. **Notch** may be seen in the superior articular facet of C7 (see Fig. 2-1B). Articular pillars of C7 extend further posteriorly than those of C6 and above. This notch is

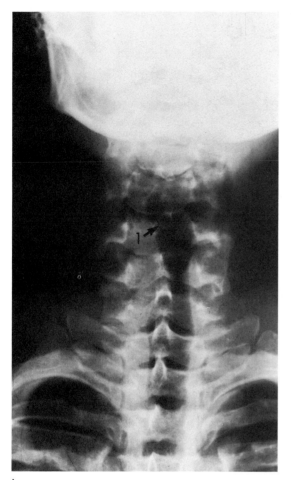

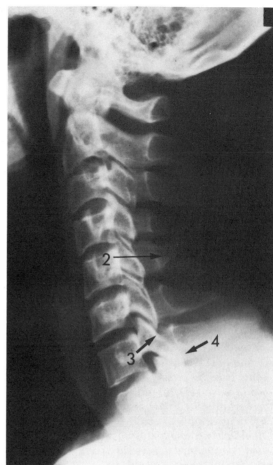

A                                                  B

**Fig. 2-6.** *Spina bifida at C5. **A.** A cleft of the spinous process is seen on the AP view **(1)**. This, too, is a normal variant. **B.** In addition, the spinous process is angled more superiorly than usual on the lateral view **(2)**. There were no associated neural abnormalities in this patient. Incidentally noted is a normal notch in the midportion of the superior facet of C7 **(3)**. The articular pillar extends further posteriorly at C7 than at higher levels **(4)**.*

**Fig. 2-7.** *Incidental findings around C1. A small process arises from both the superior and inferior aspects of the anterior C1 arch (**1** and **2**). In addition, there are two small ossicles above the C1 arch (**3**). Such separate ossicles can also occur just inferior to the arch.*

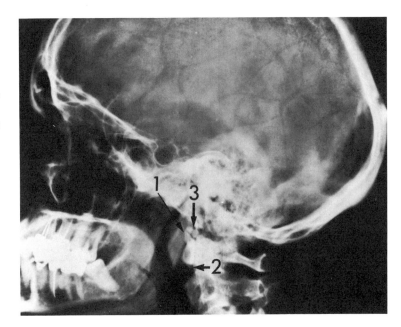

**Fig. 2-8.** *Backward tilt of odontoid. Posterior angulation of the odontoid (**1**) can be seen normally, as in this patient; however, in the presence of trauma, this finding must arouse suspicion of an odontoid fracture. Odontoid views and tomography should be obtained if there has been trauma. There is an accessory ossicle inferior to the anterior aspect of the C5 vertebral body (**2**). This may occur at various levels and is the result of incomplete fusion of the ring apophysis.*

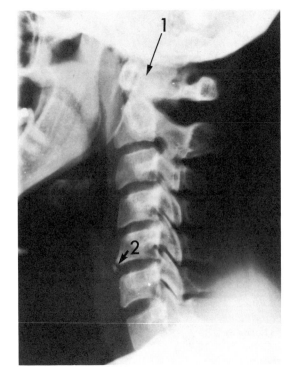

**Fig. 2-9.** *The relationship of C1 lateral masses to C2.*

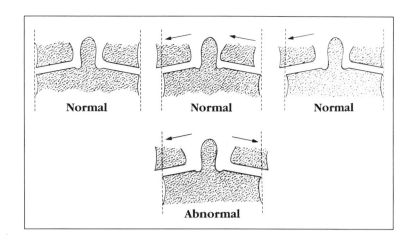

Normal     Normal     Normal

Abnormal

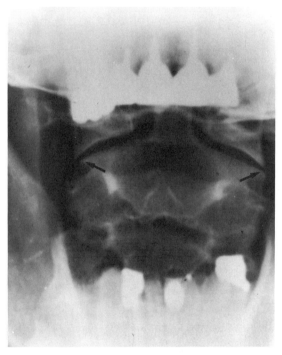

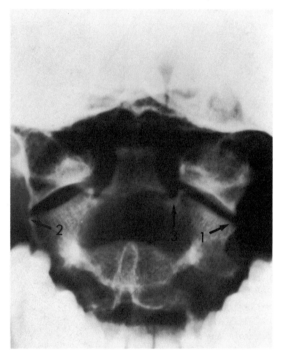

**Fig. 2-10.** *Displacement of C1 lateral masses relative to C2. Both lateral masses of C1 are displaced toward the patient's right relative to C2 (arrows). Tilting of the head in a patient with ligamentous laxity or rotation at C1–C2 may result in this normal variation. Both lateral masses of C1 are minimally displaced to the same side.*

**Fig. 2-11.** *Unilateral displacement of C1 lateral mass relative to C2. The left facet of C1 is medial to the C2 articular facet (1), while the right articular facets align normally (2). This is a normal finding caused by slight rotation. Also notable is the difference in appearance from Fig. 2-10 at the junction between the base of the odontoid and the C2 articular pillar. In this case there is a small cleft, a normal variant (3), while in Fig. 2-10 no such cleft exists.*

**2. The Cervical Spine**     **53**

**Fig. 2-12.** *Pseudosubluxation of C2 on C3. The vertebral body of C2 is anterior to C3* **(1)**. *This is a normal finding in infants and to a lesser degree in adults. It may occur to a lesser degree at C3 on C4 or at C4 on C5. The retropharyngeal* **(2)** *and infralaryngeal* **(3)** *soft tissues are widened; this is a normal variation in infants during expiration. The retropharyngeal soft tissues normally are never wider than 4 mm if the film is taken at a distance of 6 feet; however, the infralaryngeal soft tissues are quite variable in adults.*

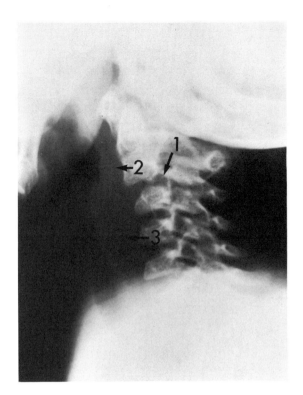

**Fig. 2-13.** *Congenital fusion of C2 and C3. The vertebral bodies are almost completely fused. A remnant of the disc space is seen anteriorly* **(1)**, *the pedicles are not fused, and the neural foramina persist* **(2)**. *The articular pillars* **(3)** *and laminae* **(4)** *appear to be completely fused, with slight separation of the spinous processes. The parts of the vertebral body and posterior arch that may fuse are variable.*

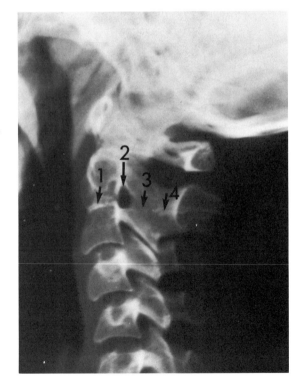

**Fig. 2-14.** *Articular pillar of C7. The posterior margin of the articular pillar of C7 extends further posteriorly (1) than the posterior margins of the articular pillars of C2–C6 (2). The apex of the lung (3) is seen anterior to T2 in this patient.*

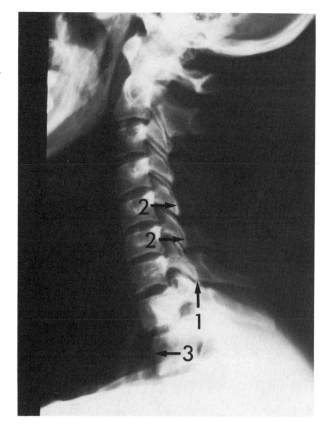

**Fig. 2-15.** *Calcified laryngeal cartilage. The laryngeal cartilages may calcify (arrow) and should not be confused with foreign bodies. Fluoroscopy and a barium swallow are helpful in differentiating the two if a foreign body is suspected.*

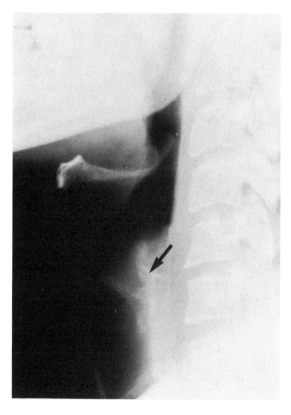

**Table 2-2.** *Is It a Fracture or a Fake Simulating a Fracture?*

|  | Fracture | Nonfracture |
|---|---|---|
| Margin of lucency | Jagged | Smooth |
|  | Sharp edges | Rounded edges |
|  | Lack of cortex (no change in density immediately adjacent to lucency of fracture) | Sclerosis of cortex (bone creates area of increased density immediately adjacent to the lucency) |
| Position | Variable | Characteristic locations of secondary ossicles, apophyses, and facet joints |
| Associated findings | Hemorrhage and soft tissue swelling | Normal soft tissues |
|  | Abnormal alignment | Normal alignment |

located at a point even with the posterior margins of the articular pillars of C6.

9. **Apex of lung** may be seen if the shoulders are low in position (Fig. 2-14).

10. **Inferior angulation** of transverse processes is a constant and identifying finding in the cervical spine; the transverse processes of the thoracic spine angulate superiorly (see Fig. 2-3).

B. Soft tissues of the neck

1. **Calcification of the laryngeal cartilages** should not be confused with foreign bodies (Fig. 2-15).

2. **Ossification of the stylohyoid ligament** is quite variable in extent (see Fig. 2-19).

3. **Retropharyngeal soft tissues** should not be thicker than about 4 mm in adults (see Fig. 2-1B).

4. **Infralaryngeal soft tissues** vary in thickness depending on age, position of the neck, and phase of respiration. They will appear thicker in very young and very old patients, especially if the neck is held in flexion. In infants and children, expiration will cause these soft tissues to appear thicker (see Fig. 2-12).

VI. **Trauma.** Fractures and subluxations

A. Findings that mimic fractures (Table 2-2):

1. Superimposed facet joint (see Fig. 2-1E).

2. Superimposed ossicles and unfused apophyses (see Figs. 2-7 and 2-8).

3. Hypertrophic bone around Luschka joints (Fig. 2-16).

4. **Caveat. If there is unexplained lucency and the edges are poorly seen, assume an acute fracture has occurred and proceed with other views, tomography, or CT for clarification.**

B. **Stability of fractures.** Several common types of injuries of the cervical spine are pictured in Figs. 2-17 through 2-28. In addition to recognition of these fractures, it is necessary to know whether they are unstable or stable (Table 2-3),

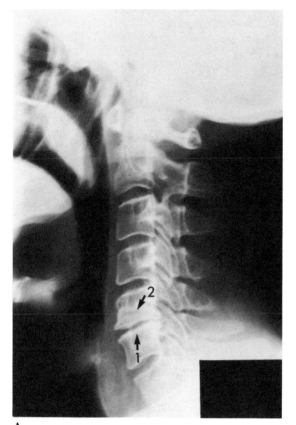

**A**

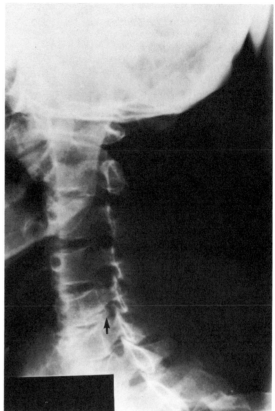

**B**

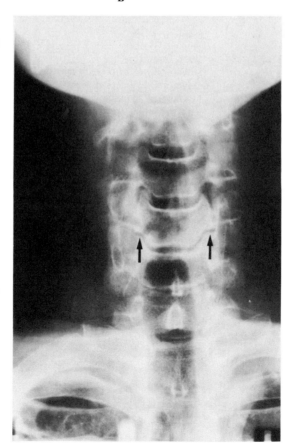

**C**

**Fig. 2-16.** *Degenerative changes at C5–C6.* **A.** *The lateral view demonstrates typical disc disease and degenerative changes at C5–C6. There are narrowing of the disc space, sclerosis of the adjacent vertebral bodies, and anterior and posterior osteophytes at this level* **(1)**. *The linear lucency across the middle third of the vertebral body* **(2)** *on the lateral view is the joints of Luschka. These joints are irregular laterally, being horizontal in orientation, and are surrounded by hypertrophic bone and sclerosis. The lucency on the lateral view is a result of "looking down the barrel" of the joints of Luschka.* **B.** *The oblique view shows osteophytes from the vertebral bodies encroaching on the C5–C6 neural foramen (arrow). Such encroachment may or may not cause pain and radicular symptoms.* **C.** *The AP view demonstrates the sclerosis and abnormal joints of Luschka at C5–C6 (arrows).*

**Fig. 2-17.** *Jefferson fracture (see Fig. 2-9). The articular facets of C1 are displaced laterally relative to both articular facets of C2 (arrows). This finding implies multiple fractures through the C1 ring. Tomograms or computed tomography may be obtained for verification.*

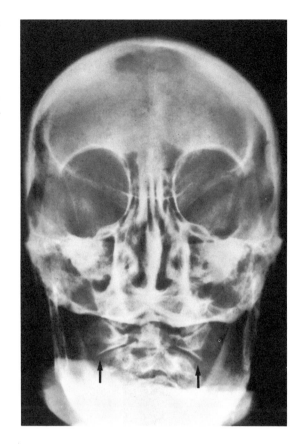

**Table 2-3.** *Stability of Cervical Spine Injuries*

| Stable injuries | Unstable injuries |
|---|---|
| Burst fracture | Jefferson's fracture |
| Unilateral posterior arch fracture | Odontoid fracture |
| Unilateral dislocation of articular pillar | Teardrop fracture |
| Fracture of articular pillar | Hangman's fracture |
| Clay-shoveler's fracture (usually stable) | Bilateral posterior arch fracture; bilateral facet dislocation |

which depends on the amount of associated ligamentous damage.

C. **Multiple fractures.** It is important to recall that about 20 percent of patients with one cervical spine fracture will have an associated second fracture in the spine.

D. **Common cervical spine injuries**
1. **Jefferson fracture** (Fig. 2-17)
   a. Consists of multiple fractures of the C1 ring.
   b. Caused by compression along axis of spine.
   c. Assumed to be present when the lateral masses of C1 are both displaced laterally relative to the articular pillars of C2. **This may be the only finding visible on plain films.**
2. **Hangman's fracture** (Fig. 2-18)
   a. Consists of bilateral fractures of the pedicles of C2
   b. Caused by hyperflexion
3. **Bilateral fractures of the laminae of C2** (Fig. 2-19)
4. **Odontoid fracture** (Fig. 2-19)
   a. Usually occurs at junction of odontoid and body of C2.
   b. May occur through odontoid or may extend into body of C2.
   c. Widened prevertebral soft tissues caused by hemorrhage is a clue.
5. **Extension teardrop fracture** (Fig. 2-20)
   a. Avulsion of anterior part of vertebral body occurs during hyperextension.
   b. Vertical lucency through vertebral body is **not** seen on AP view.
6. **Burst fracture** (Fig. 2-21)
   a. Although a stable injury, cord damage is possible because of displaced fragments.
   b. Caused by compression along axis of spine.
   c. Vertical fracture is frequently seen on AP view (in contrast to the extension teardrop fracture, in which the lucency is not seen on the AP view).
7. **Clay-shoveler's fracture** (Fig. 2-22)
   a. Consists of fracture of spinous process of C6, C7, or T1, or more than one of these vertebrae
   b. Caused by direct blow or sudden hyperflexion
   c. May be unstable if ligamentous damage is sufficient
8. **Unilateral posterior arch fracture** (see Fig. 2-18)
   a. Caused by flexion during rotation of cervical spine
   b. Is a stable injury
9. **Subluxation of C1 relative to C2** (see Figs. 2-19 and 2-30)

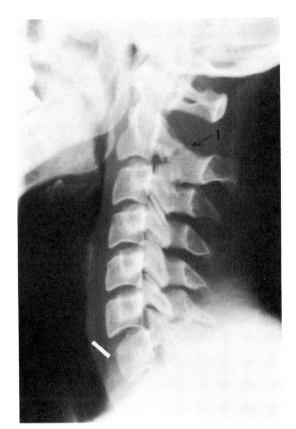

A

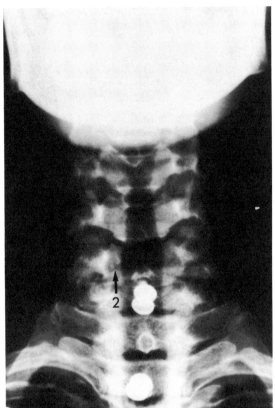

B

**Fig. 2-18.** *Hangman's fracture and unilateral fracture of C6 lamina.* **A.** *Lateral view demonstrates fracture through the pedicles and articular pillars of C2* **(1).** **B.** *AP view shows lucency through the right lamina of C6* **(2).** **C.** *Tomographic sections demonstrate the oblique fracture from the spinous process posteriorly to the articular pillar anteriorly* **(3).**

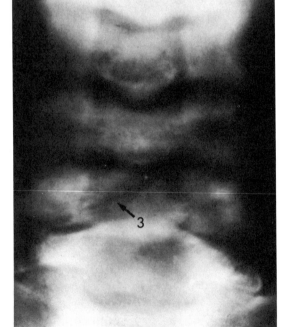

C

**Fig. 2-19.** *Odontoid fracture and bilateral fractures of C2 laminae. The lateral view demonstrates both fractures with posterior displacement and angulation of the odontoid (1). The C1 ring is displaced posteriorly, evidenced by the sudden interruption of the smooth curve of the posterior margin of the spinal canal (2). An adjunctive finding indicative of fracture is the retropharyngeal soft-tissue swelling caused by hemorrhage (3). After trauma, soft-tissue swelling implies hemorrhage with a significant amount of soft tissue damage, and perhaps an occult fracture. Incidentally noted is ossification of the stylohyoid ligament (4).*

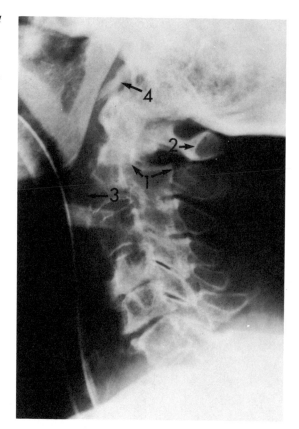

**Fig. 2-20.** *Extension teardrop fracture (arrow). The only findings in this patient are the triangular piece of bone at the inferior aspect of C2 and retropharyngeal soft tissue swelling due to bleeding.*

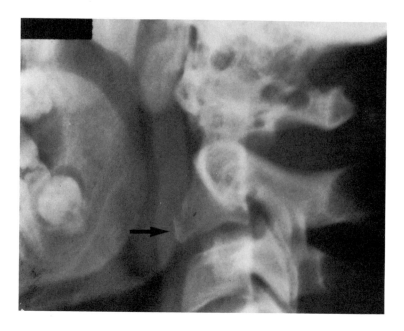

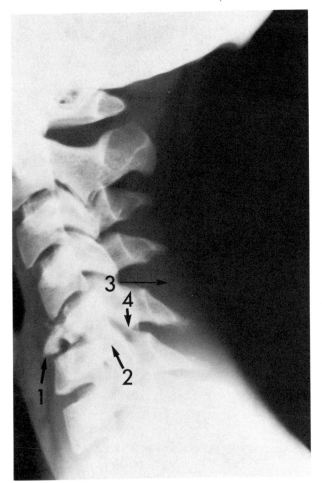

**A**

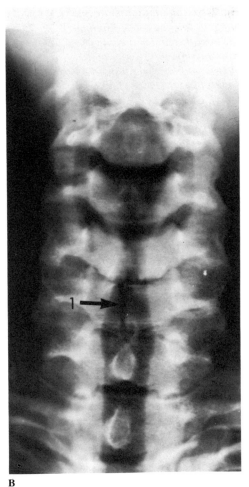

**B**

**Fig. 2-21.** *Burst fracture of C5 and C6.* **A.** *The lateral view demonstrates the triangular, anterior fragment at C5* **(1)** *and the posterior displacement of vertebral body fragments* **(2)** *into the spinal canal. The fracture of C6 is not readily apparent on this view. While a pure burst fracture may have intact ligaments and be considered stable, this patient probably encountered flexion as well as axial trauma; there is widened interspinous distance* **(3)** *and slight widening of the posterior aspect of the facet joints* **(4)** *at C5–C6. These findings imply damage to the interspinous ligament and capsular ligaments about the articular pillars; thus this injury is* **unstable.** **B.** *The AP view clearly demonstrates a vertical lucency through the C6 vertebral body* **(1)**. *This is definitely C6, since the upward directed transverse processes of T1 are a landmark. This is a minimally displaced burst fracture of C6. The vertical lucency of C5 is not as noticeable because of compression and distortion of the vertebral body. This case and that in Fig. 2-18 are good reminders that when one fracture is seen, a second fracture is more likely.*

**Fig. 2-22.** *Clay-shoveler's fracture. The spinous process of C7 is fractured (1). Flexion and extension views allow assessment of ligamentous instability. Also seen is aplasia of the spinous process of C1 (2) and prominent adenoid tissue (3); in this young patient, both are normal variations. Note: the shoulders must not be superimposed if this fracture is to be visible.*

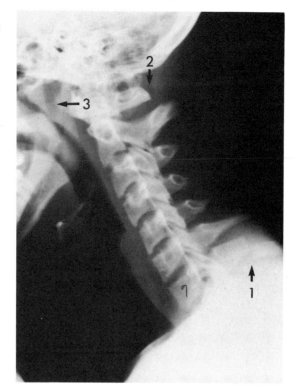

**Fig. 2-23.** *Fracture of articular pillar of C2. This patient sustained a fracture of the left articular pillar of C2. The fracture line (1) and the displacement of the lateral fragment (2) are evident.*

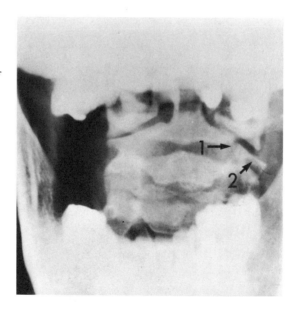

**Fig. 2-24.** *Unilateral locked facet.* **A.** *Drawing depicts the appearance of a unilateral locked facet.* **B.** *There is anterior subluxation of C5 on C6 with rotation of the upper cervical spine on the lower at this level. The rotational discrepancy is evident because the neural foramina are partially visible above C5* **(1)** *but not below C6, and because the facet joints above C5 are wide apart, while the facet joints below C6 are almost superimposed. (Above C5, one facet joint is projected over the vertebral body* **[2]**, *while the paired facet joint* **[3]** *is posterior. Below C6, the facet joints are projected over the spinal canal and are almost superimposed* **[4]**.*) The posterior margin of one of the facets of C5 remains superior and posterior to its mate at C6* **(5)**; *although subluxation is present, there is no dislocation. However, the other facet of C5 is anterior to its mate at C6* **(6)**, *implying dislocation. A "locked" facet occurs when one articular pillar dislocates anteriorly and dislocates inferior to its mate at the next lower vertebra.*

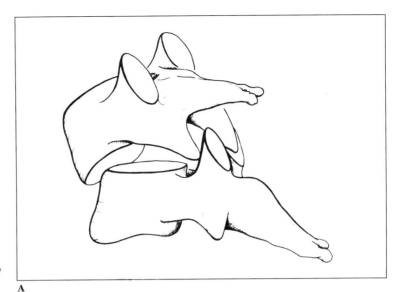

A

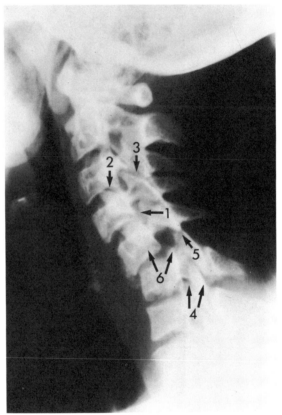

B

a. Seen with odontoid fracture or rupture or weakening of transverse atlantal (C1) ligament (trauma or rheumatoid arthritis)

b. Clue is increased distance between the anterior arch of C1 and the odontoid (greater than 3 mm in adults and 5 mm in children)

10. **Articular pillar fracture** (Fig. 2-23)

a. Caused by axial compression

b. Best seen on pillar view

11. **Unilateral locked facet** (Figs. 2-24 and 2-25)

a. Caused by flexion and rotation

b. Evidence should be sought of rotation of upper cervical spine relative to the lower cervical spine at site of injury.

(1) Facet joints appear superimposed below site of injury but separated above site of injury (lateral view).

(2) Intervertebral foramina visible above but not below site of injury (lateral view).

(3) Posterior margins of articular pillars do not align in smooth curve.

c. Articular pillar of upper vertebral body will be displaced anteriorly and inferiorly with respect to the articular pillar of the lower vertebral body ipsilaterally.

d. Scoliosis is frequently seen (AP view).

12. **Bilateral locked facets** (Fig. 2-26)

a. Caused by flexion.

b. Upper cervical spine is displaced anteriorly over the lower at the site of injury.

c. Both articular pillars of upper vertebra are anterior and inferior to articular pillars of lower vertebra.

d. Good clue is that distance between spinous processes at site of injury is widened.

e. **Caveat.** It is imperative to visualize the C7–T1 level to exclude such dislocations. Use special views if necessary.

13. **Anterior subluxation** (Figs. 2-27 and 2-28)

a. Caused by flexion.

b. Plain films may appear normal. Injury will be evident in flexion and extension views.

c. Possible findings

(1) Widening of distance between spinous processes and laminae

(2) Widening of facet joints at site of injury

(3) Visible anterior subluxation

(4) Associated fractures

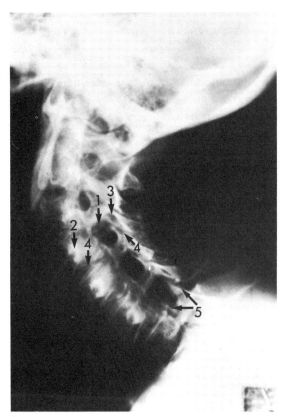

A

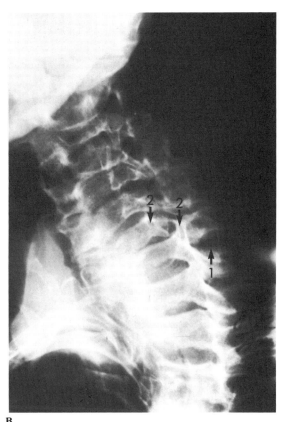

B

**Fig. 2-25.** *Unilateral locked
facet at C6–C7. This diagnosis
is difficult to establish with
scoliosis, which frequently accompanies a unilateral locked
facet.* **A.** *The lateral view does
not look typically lateral because of the rotational abnormality of the cervical spine
above the C6–C7 level. Superior
to C6–C7, the lateral view looks
like an oblique view. (The neural foramina [1], pedicles [2],
and laminae [3] are visible.)
However, C7 is seen in an almost
lateral projection. The articular
pillars above the C6–C7 level
are widely separated (4), while
they are only slightly separated
below this level (5). On one
side, the articular pillars have
become subluxed but have not
dislocated.* **B.** *The right posterior
oblique (RPO) view demon-*

*strates widening of the facet
joint of C7 on the left but no dislocation (1). Disruption of the
normally smooth alignment of
the spinous processes at this
level (2) demonstrates that the
upper cervical spine has rotated
anteriorly on the right side.*
**C.** *The left posterior oblique
(LPO) view confirms the presence of a locked articular pillar
on the right. Note: Below C7 the
right laminae and superimposed
articular pillars form a smooth
curve (1). Above this level, the
laminae are no longer seen because of the rotation; however,
the articular pillars resume a
smooth curve anterior to those
below (2).* **D.** *The AP view demonstrates the scoliosis that frequently accompanies a unilateral locked facet.*

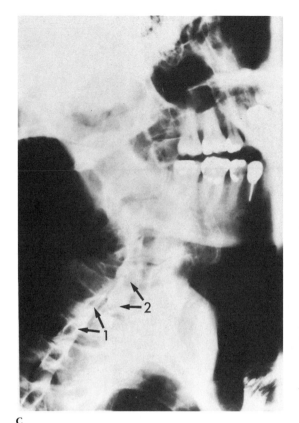

C

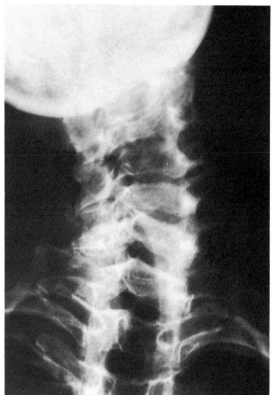

D

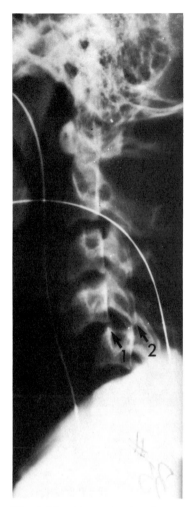

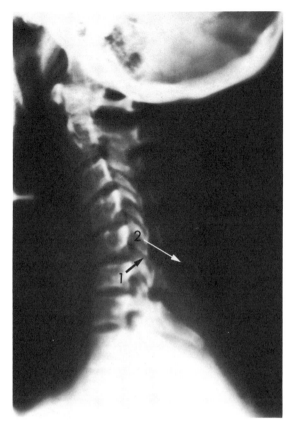

**Fig. 2-26.** *Bilateral locked facets. The lateral view clearly shows the anterior displacement of C4 on C5 (1) and that both articular pillars of C4 are locked anterior to those of C5 (2).*

**Fig. 2-27.** *Anterior subluxation. This patient demonstrates reversal of the cervical lordosis, which normally centers at C5 – C6. Above this level, the spine is in a kyphotic alignment, while below this level there is lordosis. There is no actual anterior subluxation of the vertebral body, although the posterior margins of the articular pillars of C5 are disproportionately anterior to the corresponding posterior margins of C6 when compared to other levels (1). Also, the distance between the spinous processes is too wide at this level (2). These findings lead one to suspect that an anterior subluxation has occurred, with ligamentous injury. Flexion and extension views are the next step to assess ligamentous instability.*

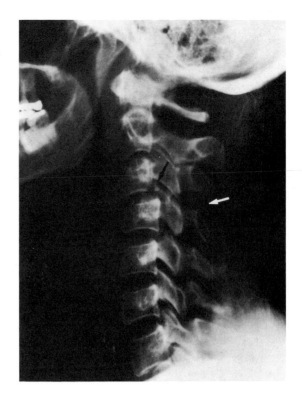

**Fig. 2-28.** *Anterior subluxation with fracture. C3 has subluxed anterior to C4. In addition, there is widening of the interspinous distance (white arrow) and an avulsion fracture from the posterior surface of C3 (black arrow).*

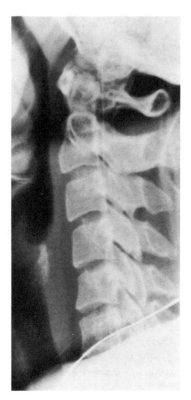

**Fig. 2-29.** *Loss of cervical lordosis. Loss of the normal lordosis, or straightening of the cervical spine, is a frequent finding due to pain and muscle spasm.*

**2. The Cervical Spine**

69

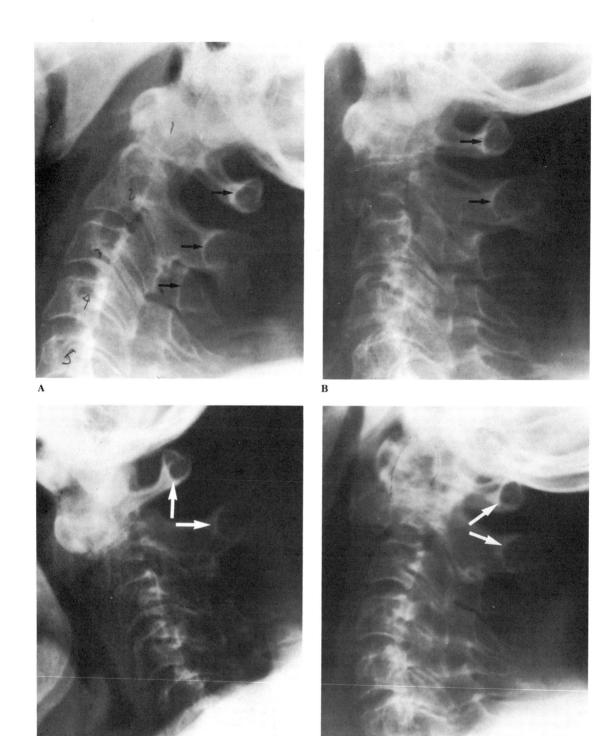

**A**

**B**

**C**

**D**

**Fig. 2-30.** *Metastatic adenocarcinoma with pathologic fracture of C2.* **A.** *The initial radiograph shows a normal relationship of C1 and C2. Note the normal alignment of the posterior margin of the spinal canal (arrows).* **B.** *Two months later, the body of C2 is destroyed. In addition, the alignment of the posterior margin of the spinal canal is abnor-* *mal, indicating anterior subluxation of the dens and C1 on the body of C2 (arrows). A pathologic fracture through the base of the odontoid or body of C2 must occur to allow this subluxation. C2 is so destroyed that no discrete fracture line is apparent. The alignment of the anterior aspect of the vertebral bodies is* *more difficult to assess but is abnormal.* **C, D.** *Flexion and extension views demonstrate the unstable nature of this injury. Again, the degree of instability is demonstrated by the anterior subluxation. This is seen by the abnormal increase in distance between the spinous processes of C1 and C2 (arrows).*

**VII. Degenerative changes** (see Fig. 2-16)

    **A. Symptoms.** Hypesthesia, numbness, cervical pain, arm pain

    **B. Findings**

        **1.** Disc space narrowing

        **2.** Osteophytes (which may encroach on intervertebral foramina)

        **3.** Sclerosis about joints of Luschka or facet joints

        **4.** Retrolisthesis (posterior displacement of upper over lower vertebra)

**VIII. Muscle spasm** (Fig. 2-29)

    **A.** Loss of normal lordotic curve (lateral view) is clue.

    **B.** May see scoliosis (torticollis) on AP view.

**IX. Tumor** (Fig. 2-30)

    **A.** May be seen in the emergency room setting because of pain.

    **B.** Lytic destruction, sclerosis, and subluxation should be sought.

    **C.** Usually caused by metastasis, frequently with a known primary carcinoma.

SELECTED READINGS

Calenhoff L, Chessare JW, Rogers LF, et al. Multiple level spinal injuries: Importance of early recognition. AJR 130:665, 1978.

Dolan, KD. Cervical spine injuries below the axis. Radiol Clin North Am 15:247, 1977.

Gehweiler JA Jr, Clark WM, Schaaf RE, et al. Cervical spine trauma: Common combined conditions. Radiology 130:77, 1979.

Gerlock AJ Jr, Kirchner SG, Heller RM, Kaye JJ. Advanced exercises in diagnostic radiology: The cervical spine in trauma. Radiology 131:628, 1979.

Harris JH Jr. Acute injuries of the spine. Semin Roentgenol 13:53, 1978.

Harris JH. *The Radiology of Acute Cervical Spine Trauma* (2nd ed.). Baltimore: Williams & Wilkins, 1987. P. 116.

Miller MD, Gehweiler JA, Martinez S, et al. Significant new observations on cervical spine trauma. AJR 130:659, 1978.

Regenbogen VS, Rogers LF, Atlaas SW, et al. Cervical spinal cord injuries in patients with cervical spondylosis. AJR 146:277, 1986.

Scher AT. Plea for routine radiographic examination of the cervical spine after head injury. S Afr Med J 51:885, 1977.

Scher AT. Anterior cervical subluxation: Unstable position. AJR 133:275, 1979.

# 3

# Thoracic and Lumbar Spine, Pelvis, and Hips

*James T. Rhea and Eric vanSonnenberg*

Chronic pain or injury are the most frequent reasons for radiographic evaluation of the thoracic and lumbar spine, pelvis, and hips. Traumatic injury to these areas frequently is associated with chest, abdominal, or other osseous injuries. These structures must not be overlooked when more vital injuries are sustained from major trauma. Evaluation must be thorough, with consideration for the total care of the patient.

   I. **Indications for examination**
      **A.** Trauma
      **B.** Pain
      **C.** Scoliosis
      **D.** Gait disturbance, radicular findings, or other neurologic abnormality
      **E.** Search of metastases
  II. **Information sought from the radiographs**
      **A.** Presence of, site, and extent of the lesion or injury
      **B.** Degree and type of displacement
      **C.** Deformity of vertebra or spinal canal
      **D.** Presence of bony fragments or foreign bodies
      **E.** Appearance of adjacent soft tissue structures
 III. **Patient movement.** Following trauma, or in the presence of unexplained pain, the patient should be moved on a **flat board** or by several people using a sheet as a **drawsheet.** Care must be taken to **avoid stressing the site of injury** to prevent further damage to the spinal cord or other soft tissues.
  IV. **Routine views and indications for further studies**
      **A.** Routine views
         **1. Thoracic spine.** Anteroposterior (AP), lateral
         **2. Lumbar spine.** AP, lateral of spine, coned lateral centered at L5–S1
         **3. Pelvis.** AP
         **4. Sacrum and coccyx.** AP, lateral
         **5. Sacroiliac joints.** Angled AP, obliques if needed
         **6. Hips.** AP, "frog lateral" (hip abducted) or true lateral
      **B.** Indications for further studies

| PROBLEM | PROCEDURE |
|---|---|
| Cannot see upper thoracic vertebral bodies on lateral view | Swimmer's view (see Fig. 2-2), tomography, or computed tomography (CT) |
| Point tenderness or persistence of symptoms over time | Coned views at various angles, tomography, bone scan,* or CT |
| Cannot see pars interarticularis or facets of lumbar spine with question of abnormality on AP or lateral films | Oblique views |
| Radicular symptoms or other signs of disc disease | Sectional imaging (CT, magnetic resonance) or myelography |
| Suspected aortic aneurysm or dissection | Ultrasound, (abdomen only), CT or angiography (chest and abdomen) |
| Cannot decide if fracture is present | Coned views, tomography, CT, bone scan |
| Suspected associated soft tissue injury: urethra, bladder, kidney, spleen, liver, pelvic hemorrhage | Urethrography, cystography, intravenous urography, liver-spleen scan, CT, ultrasound, angiography |

**V. Trauma**

    **A. Thoracic and lumbar spine trauma.** The thoracic spine is less frequently injured than the lumbar or cervical spine owing to the increased stability afforded by the ribs and alignment of the facets.

        **1. Fractures and dislocations** (Table 3-1)

            **a. Anterior compression fracture** (Fig. 3-1)

                **(1)** Accounts for **60 percent** of spinal injuries

                **(2)** Usually occurs from **T10 to L3**

                **(3)** Caused by **excessive flexion**

                **(4)** **Stable** injury, since posterior ligaments are intact

                **(5)** Frequently seen with underlying **osteoporosis** and minimal trauma

            **b. Burst fracture** (Fig. 3-2)

                **(1)** Caused by **axial compression** (e.g., fall from height).

                **(2)** **Stable** injury, ligaments intact.

                **(3)** May see **fracture of the end plate** caused by disc herniation, **fragmentation** of vertebra with **anteriorly or posteriorly displaced fragments,** or an **oblique fracture** through the vertebral body.

---

*About 50 percent of bone mineral must be destroyed by malignancy before the change is visible on plain films. A bone scan is more sensitive.

**Table 3-1.** *Stability of Thoracic and Lumbar Spine Fractures*

| Stable | Unstable |
|---|---|
| Anterior compression | Anterior dislocation of vertebra |
| Isolated unilateral dislocated facet in lumbar spine | Anterior and lateral vertebral dislocation |
| Pedicle fracture | Posterior vertebral dislocation (may be stable in flexion if mild injury) |
| Burst fracture | |
| Spinous process fracture | |
| Transverse process fracture | |

  c. **Fracture-dislocation** (Figs. 3-3 and 3-4)
    (1) **Anterior or lateral dislocation** caused by **flexion** or **flexion and rotation**
      (a) **Unstable,** with disruption of posterior ligaments and disc
      (b) **Facets** may lock
      (c) Possible **vertebral body fracture,** including body below dislocation
      (d) May **dislocate laterally** with **fracture of articular process**
    (2) **Posterior dislocation** caused by **extension**
      (a) **Unstable** if severe or **stable in flexion** if posterior ligaments intact: anterior longitudinal ligament, disc, and capsular ligaments may rupture.
      (b) **Pedicles may fracture,** leaving anterior ligament intact.
      (c) **Anterior vertebral body may fracture** instead of anterior ligament (similar to extension teardrop fracture in the cervical spine).
  d. **Spinous process fracture**
    (1) Occurs with **flexion** or a **direct blow** as an isolated finding.
    (2) Clay-shoveler's fracture if at T1.
    (3) Spinous process fracture may be a component of more severe injury (Fig. 3-4).
  e. **Transverse process fracture** (Fig. 3-5)
    (1) Usually caused by excessive **contraction of psoas muscle** or **direct blow.**
    (2) Psoas may appear enlarged, or its margin may be obliterated.
    (3) Can be confused with unfused apophysis (latter has smooth, dense margins rather than sharp edges of a fracture).
    (4) Associated with visceral (renal, spleen, liver) injuries.

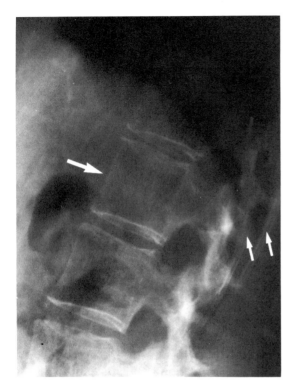

A

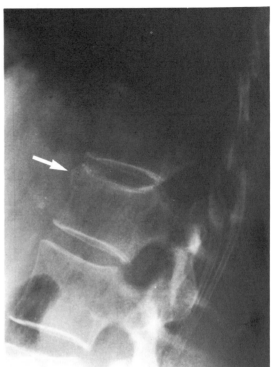

B

**Fig. 3-1.** *Anterior compression fracture. This is the most frequent injury to the thoracic and lumbar spine.* **A.** *Film obtained before the patient's fracture shows the L1 vertebra to be of normal height (single arrow). The lowermost ribs articulating with T12 help identify the level (paired arrows).* **B.** *Following injury, the fragment from the anterior superior end plate is evident (arrow). The loss of height causes surprisingly little other visible change in the vertebral body.* **C.** *A normal variation not to be confused with compression fracture, seen here in a different patient, is that the anterior height of T12 or L1 may be slightly less than the posterior height (arrows).*

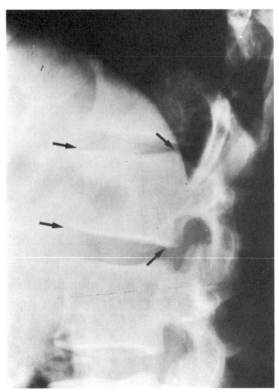

C

**Fig. 3-2.** *Burst fracture of L1 (arrow). The vertebral end plates are fractured and compressed, and there is anterior displacement of a portion of the vertebral body. Posteriorly displaced fragments (not seen here) may injure the spinal cord.*

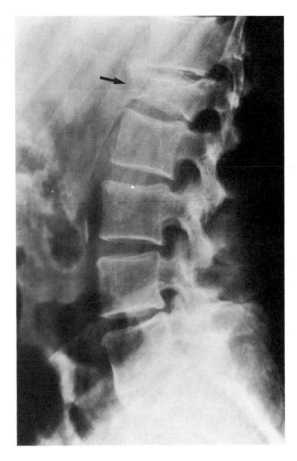

**Fig. 3-3.** *Severe fracture-dislocation—an unstable injury. The lateral displacement of T2 relative to T4 is evident by comparing the alignment of the sides of the vertebral bodies (black arrows). This abnormality should be searched for even on chest films obtained following trauma. The injury is unstable, and further spinal cord damage may result from manipulation of the patient. This patient's injury is so severe that the fractured and compressed T3 vertebra is difficult to see on this anteroposterior (AP) view. Counting the ribs (numbered) indicates the location of the remnants of T3. The junction of C7 with T1 can be identified by the upward orientation of the transverse processes of T1 compared to the horizontal or downward orientation of the transverse processes of C7 (white arrows).*

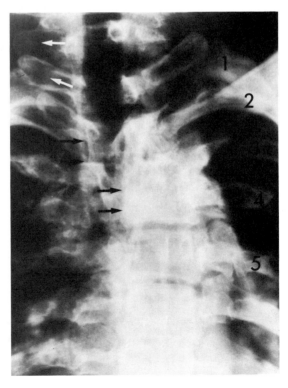

**3. Thoracic and Lumbar Spine, Pelvis, and Hips** 77

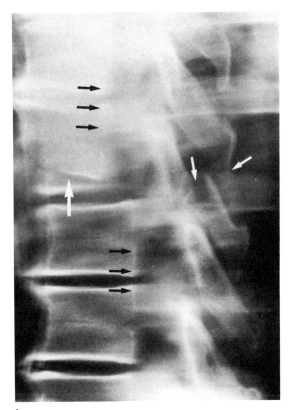

A

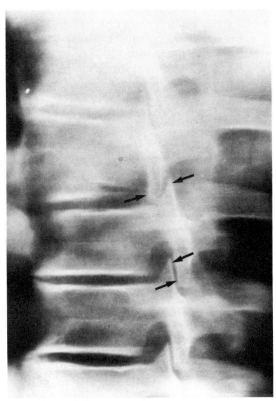

B

**Fig. 3-4.** *Extent of fracture-dislocation determined by tomography. **A.** A lateral tomographic section obtained through the middle of the thoracic vertebra shows the horizontal fracture through the vertebral body (large white arrow). The anterior displacement of the upper thoracic spine relative to the lower is seen by comparing the alignment of the posterior margins of the vertebral bodies (black arrows). A fracture through the middle of one spinous process and the superior portion of another is seen (small white arrows). **B.** A tomographic section obtained more laterally through the articular facets shows a dislocated (locked) facet at the level of the fracture (upper arrows) compared with the normal relationship of the facets below the fracture (lower arrows).*

**2. Hemorrhage** (Figs. 3-5 and 3-6)

a. Hemorrhage may be seen as **lateral displacement of paravertebral** stripe in thoracic spine.

(1) May occur as isolated finding.

(2) May be associated with thoracic spine fracture. **It is imperative to exclude potentially unstable fracture if this finding is present. Check carefully for this finding on all portable chest films in trauma.**

b. Hemorrhage may result either in enlargement of the psoas or in obliteration of its margin.

**B. Pelvic trauma**

**1. Soft tissue injury component** (Fig. 3-7)

a. **Associated injuries** occur with approximately **65 percent** of pelvic fractures.

b. **Injuries to urethra and bladder**

(1) Most frequently seen with **bilateral fractures of the anterior segment of the pelvic ring** or **wide separation of pubic symphysis**

(2) **Evaluation**

(a) **Urethrogram. A urethrogram is obtained before a Foley catheter is placed** if urethral

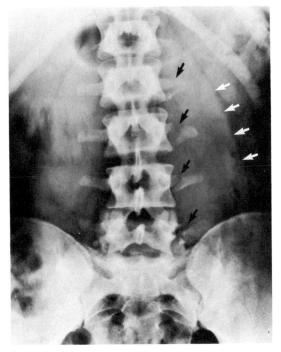

A

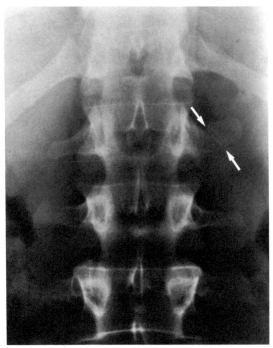

B

**Fig. 3-5.** *Transverse process fracture versus unfused apophysis.* **A.** *Several of the lumbar transverse processes have been fractured (black arrows). In addition, the psoas muscle on the side of the fractures bulges outward more than the opposite side (white arrows) because of spasm or hematoma.* **B.** *An unfused apophysis of the transverse process (arrows) has a smooth surface, rounded edges adjacent to the lucency, and a dense or white cortical margin at the edge of the lucency. Fractures have more irregular margins and acute angles at the edges of the lucent area and lack a dense cortical margin.*

injury is likely. **A Foley can transform an incomplete urethral tear into a transection.**

  (b) **Cystogram.** After the urethra is evaluated and a suprapubic or Foley catheter is in place, bladder integrity is evaluated with a cystogram.

c. **Injuries to rectum**

  (1) **Wide separation of pubic symphysis** may result in rectal tear.

  (2) **Bony fragments** may perforate the rectosigmoid colon.

  (3) To evaluate rectal tear or perforation, **Gastrografin or Hypaque enema** is indicated.

d. **Hemorrhage.** Pelvic hemorrhage can be extensive and life-threatening.

  (1) CT or ultrasound may demonstrate hematoma and is indicated if the patient is stable.

  (2) **Angiography** is indicated for diagnosis and embolic therapy when bleeding is active and the vital signs are maintained.

2. **Fractures and dislocations**

  a. **Fractures of pelvic rings** (Figs. 3-7 and 3-8)

  (1) The pelvic bones form **three rings.** The pubic and ischial bones bilaterally form the two **obturator foramina,** and the pubic, iliac, and sacral bones form the ring of the **pelvic inlet.**

**Fig. 3-6.** *Widening of the para-vertebral stripe after trauma implies hemorrhage.* **A.** *In normal patients, the paravertebral stripe is intimately applied to the vertebral bodies (black arrows). The edge of the descending aorta is more lateral and slightly oblique (white arrows); it should not be confused with the paraspinal stripe.* **B.** *Following trauma, widening of the distance between the paravertebral stripe (black arrows) and vertebral bodies indicates hemorrhage. The descending aorta is again seen (white arrows).*

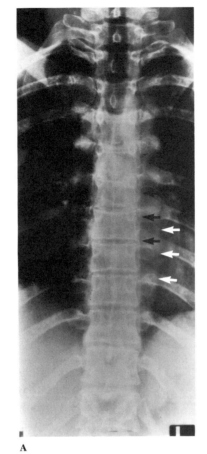

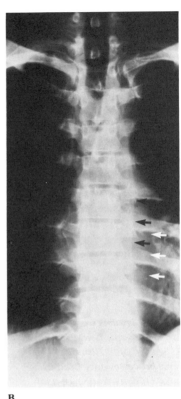

A                              B

**Fig. 3-7.** *Pelvic fractures, urethral injuries, and Foley catheters.* **A.** *Separation of the pubic symphysis should arouse concern for a tear of the urethra, bladder, or rectum. This patient has separation of the pubic symphysis (1), fracture of the right superior pubic ramus (2), fracture of the right inferior pubic ramus near its junction with the ischium (3), and separation of the right sacroiliac joint. The sacroiliac joint is not well seen on this film, but separation is suggested because the right iliac wing appears wider than the left. This appearance occurs because of posterior rotation of the iliac bone at the sacroiliac joint. Rotation of a normal patient is a*

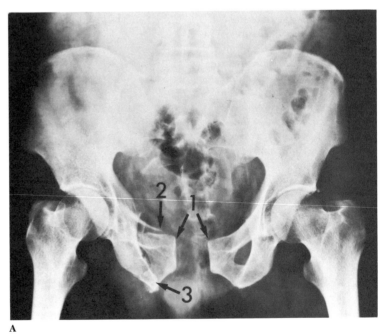

A

**Fig. 3-7** (*continued*)
*pitfall since this results in a
similar appearance.* **B.** *A urethrogram shows narrowing of
the prostatic urethra (arrows)
from hemorrhage, but no urethral tear (no extravasation of
the contrast).* **C.** *A urethrogram
performed on a different patient
with a similar injury shows extravasation of contrast (arrows),
which results from a partial
or complete tear of the urethra.
A Foley catheter should not
be inserted blindly because a
partial tear can be converted
into a complete tear. A suprapubic catheter should be placed
instead.*

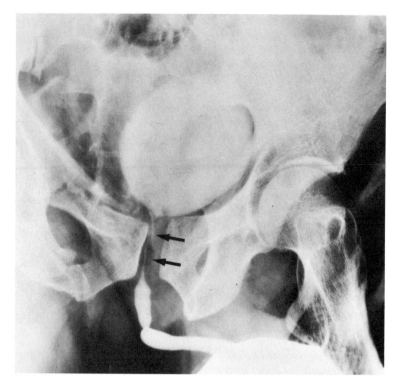

B

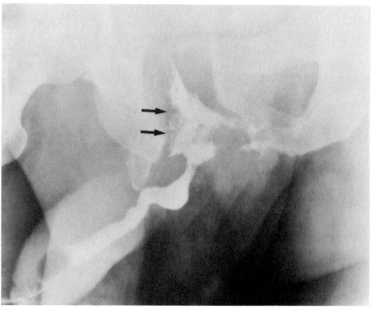

C

**Fig. 3-8.** *The pelvic ring typically fractures or separates in at least two places.* **A.** *There is separation of the pubic symphysis and left sacroiliac joint. Not only is the left pubic bone* **(1)** *higher than the right* **(2)***, there is also superior displacement of the entire left hemipelvis (note the difference in height of the hips). The left sacroiliac joint is wider than the right (black straight arrows). There is a fracture of the left ilium (black curved arrow) and avulsion fractures of both pubic bones (white arrows).* **B.** *Two subtle fractures are present near the left obturator foramen. Findings include a cortical break (straight arrow), asymmetry of the superior pubic ramus, and a line of increased density (curved arrow) representing the overlapping fractured bones adjacent to the junction of the pubic and ischial bones.*

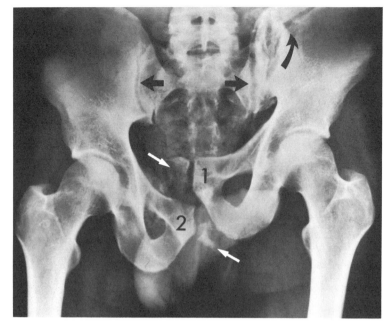

A

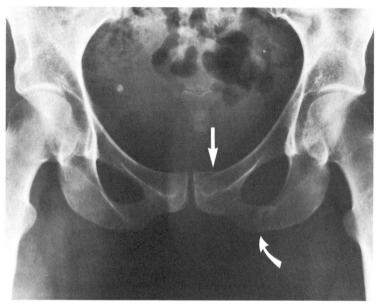

B

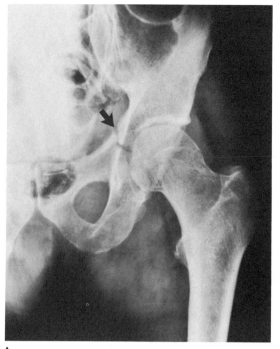

A

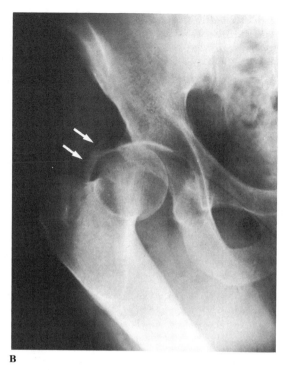

B

**Fig. 3-9.** *Acetabular fractures may be isolated or may be part of a pelvic or hip injury. A. Isolated acetabular fracture (arrow) results from force transmitted along the axis of the femoral neck or shaft. The anterior portion of the acetabulum is much thinner than the dome or posterior portion; however, the fracture site depends on the direction of force. B. Fractures of the acetabular rim usually occur posteriorly. They frequently coexist with posterior dislocation of the hip. If a posterior dislocation is seen on the AP view, but no acetabular fracture, oblique and lateral views must be obtained to exclude a fracture. In this patient with posterior dislocation of the hip, the posterior acetabular rim is fractured and displaced just above the femoral head (arrows).*

(2) While an isolated fracture of one of these bones is possible (especially with a direct blow), **usually a ring will be injured in two places,** e.g., **fracture of two bones, a fracture plus a separation of a joint** (pubic symphysis or sacroiliac joint), or **separation of the pubic symphysis and sacroiliac joint;** each constitutes the "double break" of a pelvic ring.

b. **Fractures of acetabulum** (Fig. 3-9)

    (1) These usually result from transmitted force through the femur or femoral neck.

    (2) The **hip may dislocate** anteriorly, centrally, or posteriorly.

    (3) Plain films are inadequate to detect intraarticular fragments; CT should be obtained.

c. **Isolated fracture of ilium, ischium, or pubis** (Fig. 3-10)

    (1) Usually results from a **direct blow.**

    (2) May be a **fatigue (stress) fracture** involving the **superior** or **inferior pubic ramus.** This may occur in late pregnancy.

d. **Avulsion fractures** (Fig. 3-11)

    (1) Produced by excessive muscle contraction

**Fig. 3-10.** *Isolated fracture of ischial ramus.* **A.** *While the rings of the pelvis usually fracture in more than one place, a direct blow or mild stress can result in an isolated fracture. This patient has an isolated fracture of the ischium (arrows).* **B.** *A subsequent film demonstrates the periosteal reaction that occurs with healing of the fracture (arrows). This appearance could be confused with a bone tumor without the history of prior trauma.*

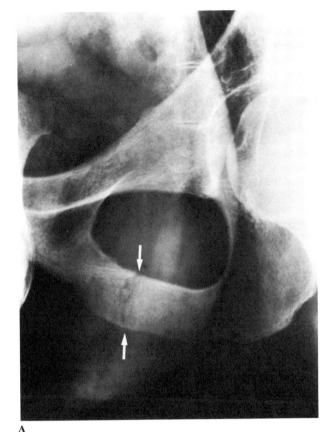

A

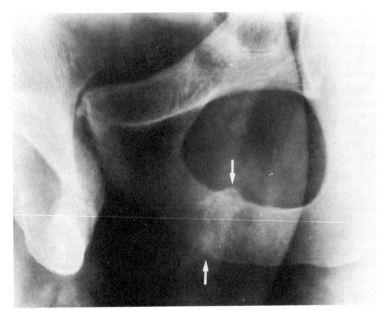

B

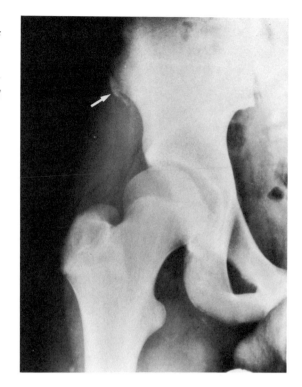

**Fig. 3-11.** *Avulsion of the anterior superior iliac spine. A sports injury frequently is the cause of this fracture (arrow). Local tenderness with the appropriate history is important in establishing the diagnosis. Comparison with radiographs of the opposite side and whether or not there is soft tissue swelling helps differentiate an apophysis.*

    (2) Location of avulsed

| fragment | Muscle involved |
|---|---|
| Anterior superior iliac spine | Sartorius |
| Anterior inferior iliac spine | Rectus femoris |
| Ischial tuberosity | Hamstrings |

  **e. Sacral and coccygeal fractures** (Fig. 3-12)

    (1) Normally there is **anterior angulation of the distal portion** of the coccyx.

    (2) **Anterior displacement of rectal gas** by associated hematoma seen on lateral view is a valuable clue that there is a fracture.

**C. Hip trauma**

  **1. Fractures** (Figs. 3-13 and 3-14)

    **a. Trochanteric fractures**

      (1) Usually occur in the elderly with external rotation and/or direct trauma.

      (2) Are extracapsular fractures that may involve the femur just distal to the lesser trochanter.

      (3) Both trochanters may or may not be involved by the fracture.

    **b. Neck of femur fractures (subcapital fractures)**

      (1) Usually occur in elderly with rotational stress

      (2) Are intracapsular fractures

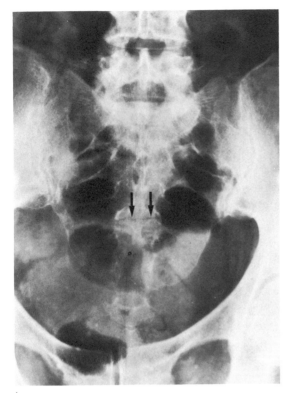

A

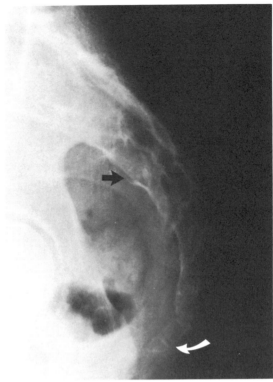

B

**Fig. 3-12.** *Sacral fractures may be difficult to visualize.* **A.** *The AP view shows a faint lucency in the midportion of the sacrum (arrows).* **B.** *The lateral view shows a cortical break anteriorly (black arrow). These subtle findings must be carefully searched for. Anterior deviation of the last two coccygeal segments is a normal finding (white arrow). The diagnosis of coccygeal fracture is difficult and must be correlated with clinical findings.*

#### c. Avulsions

(1) Greater trochanter may be avulsed by muscular pull or by direct blow.

(2) Lesser trochanter usually is a component of intertrochanteric fractures but may be an isolated finding when avulsed by the iliopsoas muscle.

### 2. Dislocations (emergency situation requiring immediate reduction) (Figs. 3-9 and 3-15)

#### a. Anterior dislocation

(1) Occurs in about 10 percent of all traumatic hip dislocations.

(2) Femoral head moves toward the obturator foramen or pubis.

#### b. Posterior dislocation

(1) May occur with fracture of the proximal femur and go unnoticed. (**Always obtain a film of the pelvis when the proximal femur is fractured.**)

(2) Posterior rim of acetabulum may be an associated fracture. **Lateral and oblique views supplement the AP film and may reveal a posterior rim fracture.**

### 3. Complications of hip fractures and dislocations (Fig. 3-16)

#### a. Late complications

(1) **Aseptic necrosis** of femoral head

    (a) Results from vascular insufficiency.

    (b) Overall incidence after dislocation is about 10 percent, but if reduction is delayed, the incidence is markedly increased (greater than 50 percent if reduction is delayed 24 hours).

(2) **Traumatic arthritis**

(3) **Myositis ossificans**

(4) **Nonunion** of fractures, which may occur with vascular compromise

#### b. Immediate complications

(1) **Sciatic nerve injury** may occur with posterior dislocations.

(2) **Loose bodies or soft tissue may be trapped** in the joint. This may result in failure of the femoral head to align properly with the acetabulum after reduction of a dislocation. A normal postreduction plain film does not exclude intraarticular fragment.

**Fig. 3-13.** *Hip fractures may be apparent or subtle radiographically. Most intertrochanteric fractures are easily seen. A nondisplaced subcapital fracture may present more difficulty in recognition. The following two fractures were "missed" initially.* **A.** *Nondisplaced subcapital fracture indicated by cortical break and faint lucency in lateral aspect of femoral neck (arrows).* **B.** *Abducted lateral view in same patient as* **A** *shows only the cortical break (arrow).* **C.** *Minimally impacted subcapital fracture in a different patient shows no cortical break. There is acute angulation between the head and neck laterally (white arrow). Also, there are faint lucencies across the femoral neck medially (small black arrows) and increased density laterally caused by impaction (large black arrow). These subtle findings indicate definite fractures.*

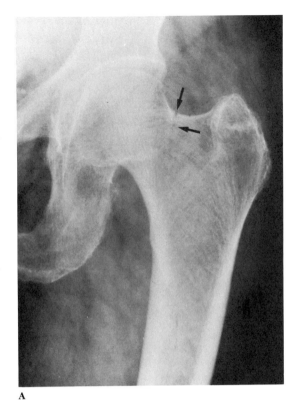

A

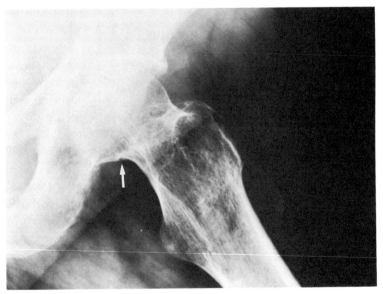

B

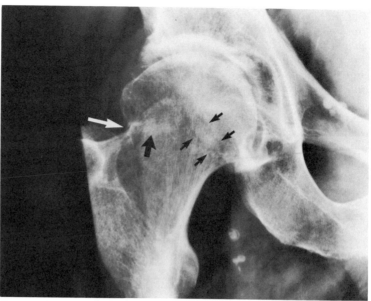

C

## VI. Nontraumatic conditions

**A. Disc disease** (Fig. 3-17). Any of the following plain film findings may be seen:

**1. Loss of height of disc space**

  **a.** Normal thoracic spine disc spaces are uniform in height.

  **b.** Normal lumbar spine disc spaces

    **(1)** Spaces from L1–L2 through L4–L5 become progressively larger.

    **(2)** Space at L5–S1 is variable and may be larger or smaller than L4–L5.

  **c.** Loss of height of disc space may not correlate with symptoms.

**2. Adjacent sclerosis** of vertebral body end plates

**3. Small anterior osteophytes**

  **a.** Arise 1 to 2 mm from the end plate

  **b.** Are oriented perpendicularly to vertical axis of vertebra

**4. Mild spondylolisthesis or retrolisthesis** (anterior or posterior displacement of upper vertebral body on lower)

  **a.** Caused by ligamentous laxity associated with decrease in height of disc

  **b.** Usually occurs in lumbar area

**5. Vacuum phenomenon** (gas within the disc space—sometimes associated with symptoms)

**6. Disc calcification**

**Fig. 3-14.** *Avulsion of femoral trochanters may be isolated findings.* **A.** *Avulsion of greater trochanter (arrow) and* **B.** *avulsion of lesser trochanter (arrow) in a different patient require casting and immobilization, respectively. These fractures may have serious sequela if not diagnosed and treated correctly.*

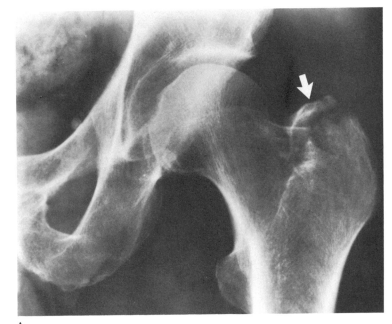

A

B

**Fig. 3-15.** *Bilateral hip disloca-*
*tion. The right hip is dislocated*
*anteriorly toward the obturator*
*foramen. In addition, there are*
*fractures through the acetabu-*
*lum, pubic, and ischial bones*
*(arrows). The left hip is dislo-*
*cated posteriorly and the pos-*
*terior rim of the acetabulum is*
*fractured. Bilateral hip disloca-*
*tion occurs in patients who had*
*their legs crossed in an automo-*
*bile accident.*

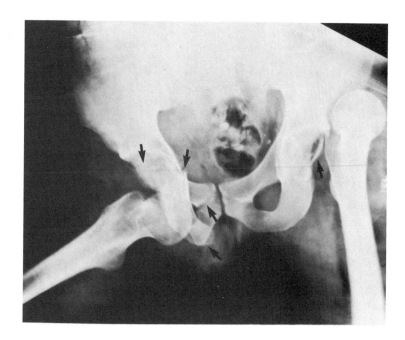

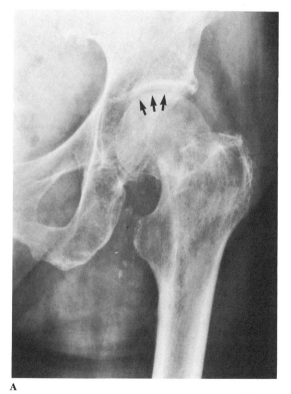

A

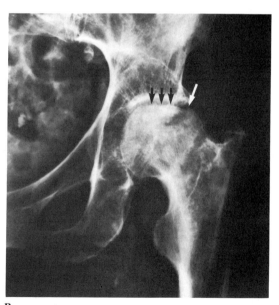

B

**Fig. 3-16.** *Aseptic (avascular)*
*necrosis of femoral head. A. The*
*earliest finding in aseptic necro-*
*sis is a thin, faint rim of lucency*
*in the immediate subcortical*
*area (arrows). At this stage, the*
*dead bone may appear slightly*
*denser than the adjacent viable*
*bone, which becomes somewhat*
*osteoporotic. B. Later, the in-*
*volved bone undergoes compres-*
*sion; note the break in the cortex*
*(white arrow) and flattening of*
*the involved portion of the head*
*(black arrows).*

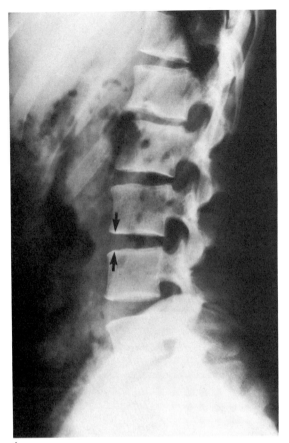

A

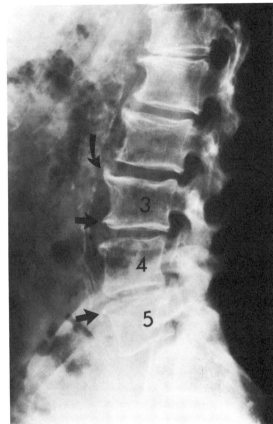

B

**Fig. 3-17.** *Radiographic findings of disc disease. A. In the normal lumbar spine, the disc spaces get progressively wider from L1–L2 through L4–L5. The space at L5–S1 is variable normally; it may be either wider or more narrow than the space at L4–L5. The width of the disc space should be assessed at the anterior portion (arrows). B. In this patient, the disc spaces at L3–L4 and L4–L5 are narrowed. (Vertebrae are numbered.) Osteophytes resulting from protrusion of the disc also are characteristic (straight arrows). They arise 1 to 2 mm from the edge of the end plate and are perpendicular to the anterior border of the vertebra. Osteophytes from degenerative disease differ—they arise at the end plate and curve toward the adjacent vertebra (curved arrow).*

**B. Degenerative joint disease** (Fig. 3-17)

  **1. Osteophytes**

    **a.** Arise at edge of end plate of vertebral body

    **b.** Curve toward adjacent vertebral body

    **c.** Usually seen anteriorly or laterally

  **2. Sclerosis and hypertrophic bone** (sometimes seen about facet joints)

  **3. Narrowing of facet joints**

  **4. Vacuum phenomenon** in the disc

**C. Osteomyelitis** (Fig. 3-18)

  **1. Staphylococcus aureus** is the most common organism. Tuberculosis, gram-negative organisms, and fungi may be seen.

  **2. Radiographic findings**

    **a. Loss of height of disc space** from disc destruction

    **b. Destruction** of end plates and cancellous bone of vertebra

    **c. Involvement of both vertebral bodies** adjacent to disc

    **d. Pathologic anterior compression** of vertebral body, e.g., gibbous deformity of tuberculosis

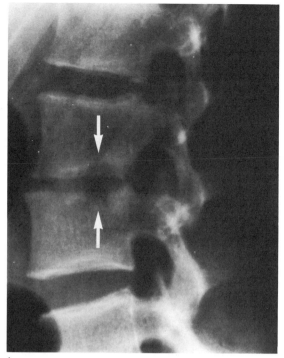

A

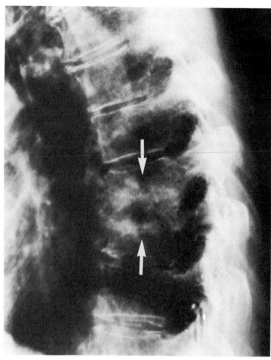

B

**Fig. 3-18.** *Osteomyelitis tends to start in the disc space. A. This example of early osteomyelitis shows narrowing of the disc space, roughening and erosion of the vertebral end plates, and faint lytic destruction and adjacent sclerosis of the contiguous vertebrae (arrows). B. In this more advanced case, the disc space is almost completely destroyed, and there is more lytic destruction and sclerotic reaction of the adjacent vertebrae (arrows).*

    **e. Reactive sclerosis** of vertebral body (occurs subacutely or chronically)

    **f. Ivory vertebra** (homogeneous sclerosis of vertebral body) seen chronically, but rare

    **g. Paraspinal mass** possible, especially in tuberculosis

    **h. Kyphosis or scoliosis**

**D. Neoplasm** (Figs. 3-19, 3-20, and 3-21)

  **1. Metastases**

    **a. Most frequent** bone neoplasm

    **b. Appearance**

      **(1) Lytic.** Thyroid, kidney, lung, untreated breast

      **(2) Mixed lytic and sclerotic.** Breast, lung

      **(3) Sclerotic.** Gastrointestinal tract, urinary bladder, prostate

  **2. Radiographic findings**

    **a. Destruction** of the pedicle of vertebral body as an isolated finding with metastasis.

    **b. Homogeneous or mottled sclerosis** of vertebra; ivory vertebra possible, but rare.

    **c. Homogeneous or mottled lytic destruction** of vertebra.

    **d. Paraspinal mass** caused by soft tissue involvement with tumor.

    **e. Periosteal reaction** possible.

**Fig. 3-19.** *Metastatic breast carcinoma: change in bony mineralization. Breast carcinoma may be either lytic or sclerotic in appearance. In this case, there is diffuse involvement of all the visualized bones with a mixed sclerotic and lytic appearance. Tumor involving bone inevitably alters the pattern of mineralization; this may occur rather late in the course of the disease.*

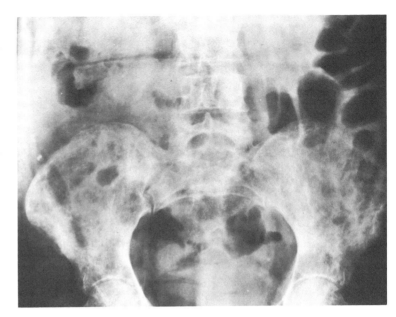

**Fig. 3-20.** *Chondrosarcoma: expansion of bone. The appearance of primary bone tumors is extremely variable. In this case, there is expansion of the bone as well as lytic destruction. The transition from normal to abnormal bone (arrow) is poorly defined. This indistinct zone of transition favors a malignant over a benign lesion.*

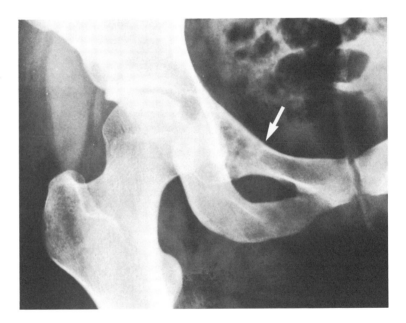

**Fig. 3-21.** *Neurofibromatosis: pressure erosion of bone from adjacent tumor. The film shows widening of neural foramina (small arrows) as well as erosion of the posterior aspect of L4 (large arrows) because of the slowly growing neurofibromata. Any pathologic process capable of placing pressure on the bone may cause erosion.*

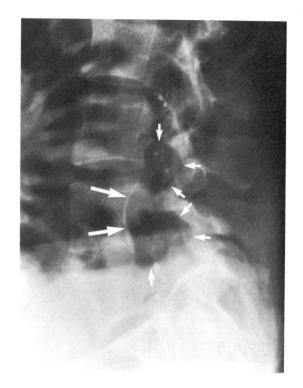

**Fig. 3-22.** *Spondylolysis and spondylolisthesis. Spondylolysis is seen as a lucent defect in the pars interarticularis (piece of bone between the superior and inferior facets [large white arrows]). Compare to the normal vertebra above (small white arrows). In addition, spondylolisthesis (anterior displacement of the upper vertebra relative to the lower) is seen (black arrows).*

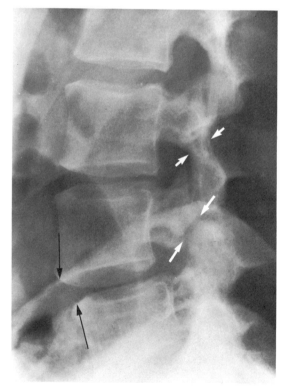

**3. Thoracic and Lumbar Spine, Pelvis, and Hips** 95

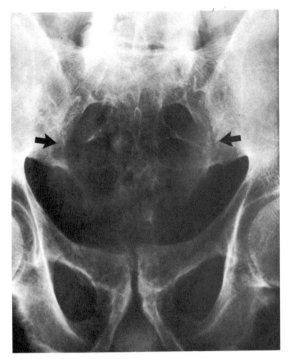

A

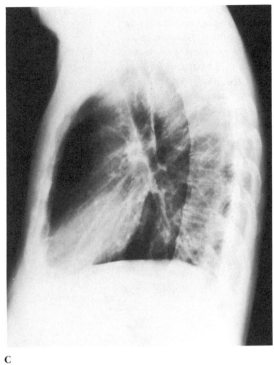

C

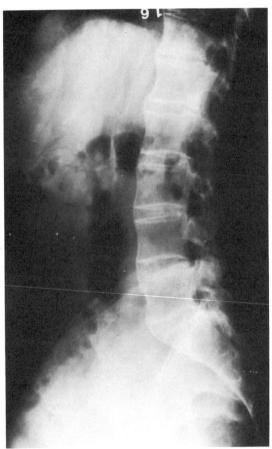

B

**Fig. 3-23.** *Ankylosing spondylitis.* **A.** *Fusion of the sacroiliac joints is seen in this patient with advanced disease (arrows).* **B.** *Calcification of the spinal ligaments results in a smooth, undulating calcific link between vertebrae.* **C.** *In the thoracic spine, the calcification of the ligaments is not as apparent, but the anterior aspects of the vertebrae appear squared-off or too straight compared with the normal, slight convexity.*

**Fig. 3-24.** *Aortic aneurysm may cause vertebral erosion. T12, L1, and L2 demonstrate anterior erosion (arrows). The finding is nonspecific; the irregularity of the borders might suggest osteomyelitis and erosion from an adjacent abscess. Back or abdominal pain may be the presenting finding with aortic aneurysm.*

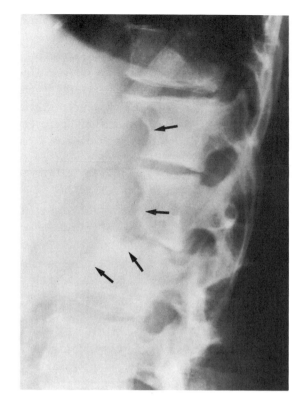

  **f. Pathologic anterior compression or dislocation** of vertebra.

  **g. Pressure erosion of vertebral body** or **neural arch.**

  **h. Focal area of sclerosis,** especially in neural arch with osteoid osteoma.

  **i. Striated trabecular pattern** characteristic of benign hemangioma.

  **j. Kyphosis or scoliosis** possible.

 **E. Spondylolysis and spondylolisthesis** (Fig. 3-22)

  **1. Occurrence**

   **a.** May occur together or separately.

   **b.** Unilateral spondylolysis (defect in pars interarticularis) occurs in about 5 percent of adults.

   **c.** Spondylolisthesis occurs in lower lumbar spine in about 3 percent of adults.

   **d.** May or may not be associated with symptoms.

  **2. Radiographic findings**

   **a.** Defect (lucency) is seen in pars interarticularis on lateral and/or oblique views.

   **b.** Special angled oblique view better visualizes the facet joints and pars interarticularis of L5.

   **c.** Narrowing of disc space and bony sclerosis may be seen with isolated spondylolisthesis.

### 3. Classification of spondylolisthesis

    **a. First degree.** One-fourth or less of vertebral body width displacement

    **b. Second degree.** One-fourth to one-half of vertebral body width displacement

    **c. Third degree.** One-half to three-fourths of vertebral body width displacement

    **d. Fourth degree.** Greater than three-fourths of vertebral body width displacement

## F. Sacroiliitis (Fig. 3-23)

### 1. Etiology

    **a. Bilateral symmetric involvement.** Psoriasis, rheumatoid arthritis, inflammatory bowel disease, ankylosing spondylitis, Reiter's syndrome

    **b. Unilateral or asymmetric involvement.** Psoriasis, infection, gout, Reiter's syndrome

### 2. Radiographic findings

    **a. Bone erosions**

    **b. Sclerosis**

    **c.** Early **widening** of sacroiliac joint

    **d.** Later **narrowing** and finally **fusion** of sacroiliac joint

## G. Aortic aneurysm (Fig. 3-24)

**1.** Back pain may be the primary complaint.

**2.** Scalloping (pressure erosion) of the anterior aspect of the vertebral body rarely can be seen.

**3.** Associated soft tissue calcification anterior to the lumbar spine may demonstrate the aneurysm.

**SELECTED READINGS**

Abel MS. Jogger's fracture and other stress fractures of the lumbosacral spine. Skeletal Radiol 13:221, 1985.

Federle MP, Brant-Zawadzki M. *Computed Tomography in the Evaluation of Trauma.* Baltimore: Williams & Wilkins, 1986.

Gehweiler JA Jr, Daffner RH. Low back pain: The controversy of radiologic evaluation. AJR 140:109, 1983.

Gehweiler JA Jr, Osborne RL Jr, Becker RF. The radiology of vertebral trauma. Vol. 16, Monographs in Clinical Radiology series. Philadelphia: Saunders, 1980. P. 459.

Gellad FE, et al. Pure thoracolumbar dislocation: Clinical features and CT appearance. Radiology 161:505, 1986.

Harris JH. Radiographic evaluation of spinal trauma. Orthop Clin North Am 17:75, 1986.

Jelsma RK, Kirsch PT, Rice JF, et al. Radiographic description of thoracolumbar fractures. Surg Neurol 18:230, 1982.

Keene JS, Goletz TH, Lilleas F, et al. Diagnosis of vertebral fractures. J Bone Joint Surg 64A:586, 1982.

Rogers LF. *Radiology of Skeletal Trauma.* New York: Churchill Livingstone, 1982.

Sartoris DJ, Clopton P, Nemcek A, et al. Vertebral-body collapse in focal and diffuse disease: Patterns of pathologic processes. Radiology 160:479, 1986.

Scavone JG, Latshaw RF, Weidner WA. Anteroposterior and lateral radiographs: An adequate lumbar spine examination. AJR 136:715, 1981.

# 4 The Extremities

*James T. Rhea and Eric vanSonnenberg*

Before obtaining x-rays of the extremities, a detailed history and physical examination will increase diagnostic yield and reduce the amount of radiation the patient is exposed to. Knowledge of the mechanism of injury will help the physician determine the type of injury; knowledge of the sites of swelling and tenderness will indicate the location of a fracture or dislocation. High-yield, coned-down views, tangential films, or special radiographs for specific locations are obtained expeditiously. This eliminates unnecessary radiographs.

The minimal radiographic examination in suspected extremity injury consists of **two views** taken 90 degrees apart, e.g., anteroposterior (AP) and lateral. **A fracture or dislocation may be elusive, showing up on one view only** (Fig. 4-1). Some fractures may not be seen on the initial x-ray series. If symptoms persist, the original "negative" radiographic examination should not lead to a false sense of security. **Repeat examination** in 10 to 14 days may demonstrate an **initially occult fracture.**

Innumerable obvious fractures and dislocations exist, and a plethora of eponyms is associated with them. Descriptions of these are not included in this chapter. Rather, the structure and focus of this section will consist of (1) guidelines necessary to diagnose a fracture in any bone, particularly in difficult cases, and (2) injuries that are common but specifically troublesome to diagnose radiographically. The second section is grouped by anatomic site. The final sections of this chapter include pertinent information on infection, arthritis, and foreign bodies in the extremities.

Several specific aids are helpful for diagnosis of extremity injuries:

1. **Comparison films of the normal side**—these may demonstrate contralateral and symmetric normal variants, clarifying questionable findings.
2. Use of a **bright light** is particularly valuable in visualizing the soft tissues, specifically **tissue swelling and joint effusion,** often **clues to fractures.**
3. Foreign bodies or gas in soft tissues must be searched for—bright light may help here also.
4. Cortical margins are frequently seen to better advantage with a bright light on overexposed (dark) films.

**Fig. 4-1.** *Fracture seen only on lateral view.* **A.** *The anteroposterior (AP) view in this case is deceptively normal. A "normal" single view does not exclude a fracture.* **B.** *The fracture is obvious on the lateral view (arrow).*

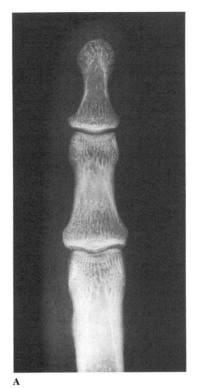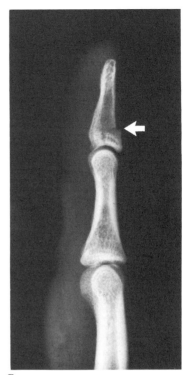

A                                                    B

**Fig. 4-2.** *Characteristic features of fractures include lucency of fracture line (1), edge of adjacent bone sharply defined (2), and acute pointed angle at the ends of the fracture (3).*

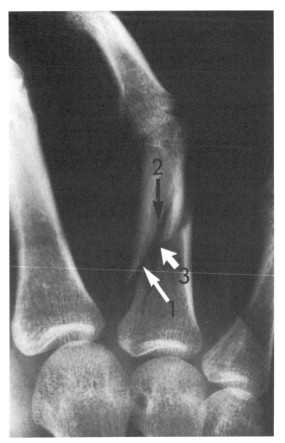

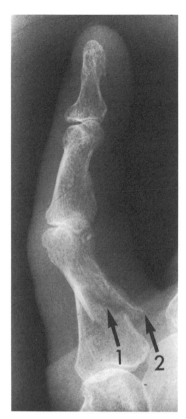

**Fig. 4-3.** *Healing fracture. Note, in comparison with Fig. 4-2, that the edges of the fracture are less sharply defined and are fuzzy (1). The ends of the fractures are rounding off (2). This fracture is 1 week old.*

**Caveat. On underexposed (light) films, nondisplaced fractures can be missed. A film is underexposed if the trabecular pattern of the bone cannot be seen.** Radiographs should be repeated if technically suboptimal.

### I. General approach to fractures

A. **Recognition of fractures. Features of acute fractures** include the following (any of which should suggest a fracture):

1. **Well-defined lucency** across the bone (Fig. 4-2).

2. **Sharp edge** of bone at the fracture site (Fig. 4-2).

3. **Pointed angle** of the bone adjacent to the fracture site in an **acute** fracture (Fig. 4-2). (**Healing** fracture resorbs bone at the fracture edge; it appears ill-defined instead of sharp. The angle at the edge of the fracture becomes rounded with time, as in Fig. 4-3.)

4. **Lack of definition of the bone cortex** at the fracture site may be the only sign of fracture and may be subtle (Fig. 4-4). The finding helps differentiate acute fractures from old ununited avulsion fractures and from secondary ossicles; the latter have sharp, circumferential cortical bone.

5. **Acute angulation, discontinuity,** or a **"bump"** in the bony cortex (Figs. 4-5, 4-6, 4-7, 4-8). The normal cortex is straight, smoothly curved, or rounded. Sudden abrupt change in angulation of the cortical edge indicates presence of a fracture. The classic example is the "torus" or "buckle fracture" (Fig. 4-8).

6. **Trabecular lucency and distortion** (see Figs. 4-5 and 4-7). This may be the only finding of a subtle fracture. The normal well-organized bony trabeculae become disorganized across the bone; this results in a faint, poorly defined lucency representing the fracture.

7. **Zone of increased density** is seen if the fracture fragments overlap or are impacted (see Figs. 4-5 and 4-6).

B. **Findings that mimic fractures**

1. **Secondary ossicles** (Fig. 4-9). These have characteristic locations and are circumferentially smooth and well corticated.

2. **Soft tissue folds** (Fig. 4-10). These may mimic the lucency of a fracture. However, the clue to a fold is that it inevitably extends off the bone into the adjacent soft tissues.

3. **Vascular grooves** (Fig. 4-11). These occur in characteristic locations, course at characteristic angles to the bony cortex, are not as lucent as acute fractures, and have slightly rounded margins at the corticated edge of the lucency.

**Fig. 4-4.** *Characteristic features of fractures. This avulsion fracture from the triquetrum lacks cortex along the inferior edge of the avulsion and at the donor site of the triquetrum (1). Note the cortical density surrounding the intact normal bones (2).*

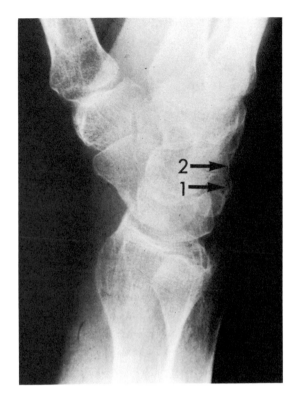

**Fig. 4-5.** *Features of fracture: subtle Colles' fracture. There is slight discontinuity of the radial cortex (1) as well as a narrow zone of sclerosis (3). These findings may be normal in adults as a result of the epiphyseal remnant. (Compare with Figs. 4-22 and 4-23.) However, there is also trabecular lucency both transverse and parallel to the axis of the radius (2) and a fracture of the ulna styloid (curved arrow).*

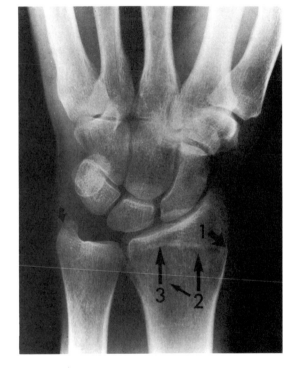

104

**Fig. 4-6.** *Characteristic features of fractures: radial head fracture. Both AP (A) and lateral (B) views demonstrate an abrupt angulation of the cortex of the radial head (1). In addition, there is a faint zone of sclerosis (2) caused by impaction and a joint effusion indicated by elevation of the posterior fat pad (3). Following trauma, an elbow joint effusion in adults implies a radial head fracture even if it is not seen. A follow-up film in 10 to 14 days may show a fracture that was not initially apparent.*

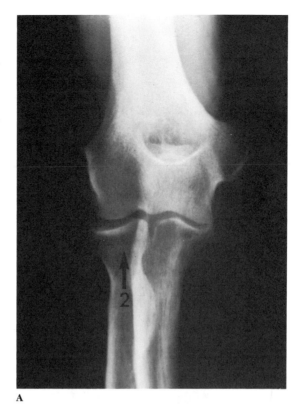

A

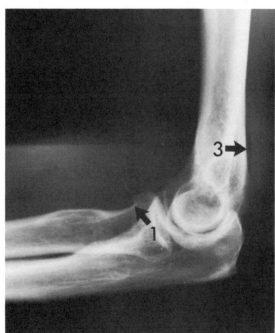

B

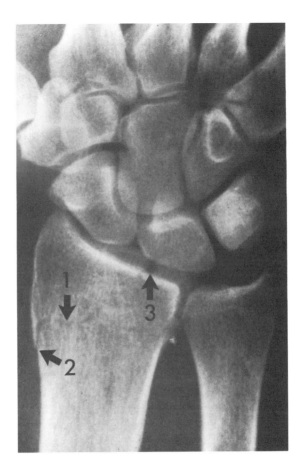

**Fig. 4-7.** *Characteristic features of fractures: Colles' fracture. No clearly defined line of fracture is visible. However, trabecular lucencies (1), a cortical break (2), and faint lucency at the articular surface (3), indicate the presence of fracture.*

    4. **Bipartite patella** (Fig. 4-12).

    5. **Epiphyses** (Fig. 4-13).

C. **Findings that indicate fractures** when actual fracture is not visible:

    1. **Fat-fluid level** in the suprapatellar knee bursa on an upright or cross-table lateral view implies a tibial plateau fracture (Fig. 4-14).

    2. **Elbow effusion** following trauma implies a radial head fracture in adults (see Fig. 4-6).

    3. **Soft tissue swelling and loss of normal fat planes** in the soft tissues demands careful examination of the underlying bone for a fracture. These findings are nonspecific, however. If a fracture is suspected but not visible on initial radiographs, a follow-up film in about 10 days should demonstrate the fracture, due to bony resorption.

D. **Situations with high likelihood of second fracture or dislocation** (Fig. 4-15). In the extremities, the paired bones (the tibia and fibula and the radius and ulna) are connected by strong interosseous membranes. As a result, force sufficient to fracture one bone frequently will fracture or dis-

**Fig. 4-8.** *Forearm fracture (torus fracture). This child fractured the distal radius. The major radiographic finding is the cortical "bump" seen on both sides of the bone on the AP view* **(A)** *and on the anterior surface of the radius on the lateral view* **(B)** *(arrows). The term "buckle fracture" has been applied to this appearance.*

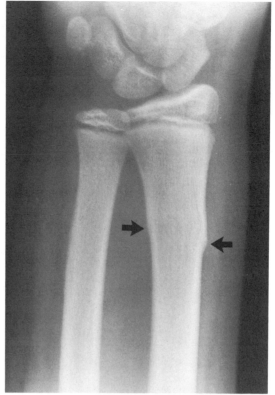

A

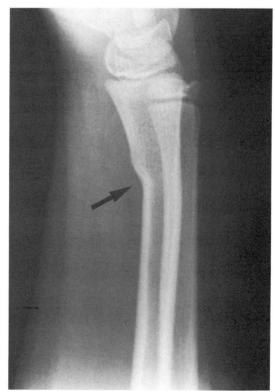

B

4. The Extremities

**Fig. 4-9.** *Characteristics of secondary ossicles (normal variants). **A.** This normal hand demonstrates a smoothly rounded ossicle (arrow) at the metacarpophalangeal joint of the thumb. There is a faint cortical rim surrounding the ossicle. **B.** A normal ankle shows an ossicle (arrow) posterior to the talus. Ossicles occur at various locations, but similar features apply to all.*

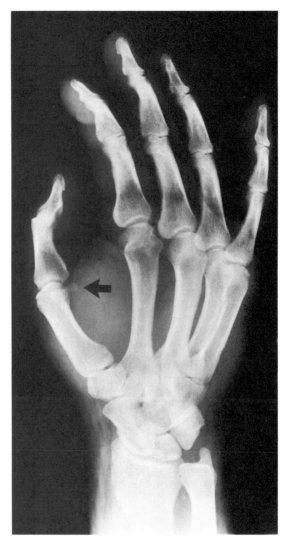

A

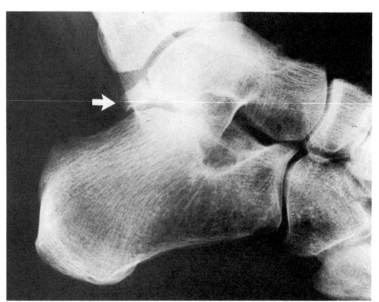

B

**Fig. 4-10.** *Skin fold versus fracture. This skinfold is caused by soft tissue swelling of the palmar surface of the hand, which superimposes over the metacarpals (arrows). The skinfold extends beyond the bone, a tip-off that the appearance is the result of "superimposition of shadows" rather than a fracture.*

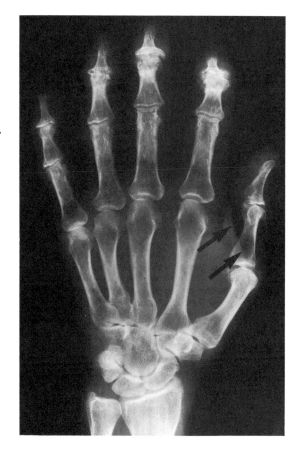

**Fig. 4-11.** *Characteristics of normal vascular channels versus fractures.* **A.** *Vascular channel in phalanx.* **B.** *Vascular channel in proximal femur. These channels are not lucent enough for fractures, given their width, and the cortex at the end of the channel (arrows) is smoothly rounded. There is no adjacent soft tissue swelling, and the locations of the channels are characteristic in each bone.*

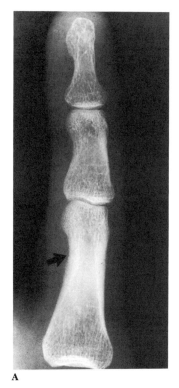

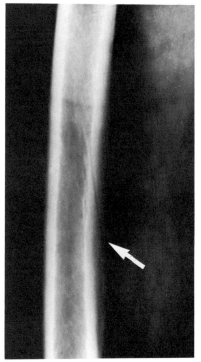

A        B

**Fig. 4-12.** *Bipartite patella, a normal variation. This normal variation occurs at the upper lateral aspect of the patella (arrow). The bipartite patella has smooth edges that are rounded on both sides of the lucency. A fracture may occur here; when in doubt, radiographic comparsion with the uninjured side is indicated.*

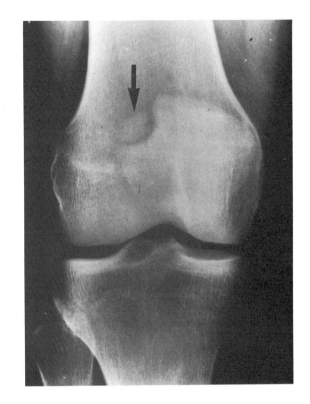

locate the other. If both fractures occur at the same joint, they will usually be seen (e.g., fracture of both medial and lateral malleoli at the ankle). However, the second fracture may occur at the opposite end of the paired bones. For example, with an ankle fracture, there may be an associated proximal fracture as well. Similarly, a fracture of the wrist or elbow may be associated with a fracture or dislocation at the opposite end of the forearm.

## II. Specific extremity injuries

### A. Shoulder

1. **Acromioclavicular separation** (Fig. 4-16)

   a. Types

   (1) **Grade I.** Sprain, no radiographic findings.

   (2) **Grade II.** Film with patient holding weights shows vertical separation of acromion from clavicle of less than full width of the clavicle.

   (3) **Grade III.** Film with or without weights shows vertical separation by more than the width of the clavicle.

   **Caveat.** Measure separation based on distance between the **inferior** margin of the acromion and **inferior** margin of the clavicle. Superior margins may not "line up" normally.

**Fig. 4-13.** *Characteristics of epiphyses.* **A.** *In patient A, the epiphyses have not fused. The edges are rounded, and the distance of the epiphyseal ossification center from the rest of the bone is variable and decreases with time. A good way to assess the integrity of an epiphyseal center is to obtain a comparison view of the opposite side. Epiphyses often form at several centers and appear fragmented, as does the trochlear epiphysis in this patient (arrow).* **B.** *In patient B, the olecranon epiphysis appears to have partially closed. The edges are rounded, and there is increased density adjacent to the epiphysis at this stage (arrow). Fractures will not have this thin line of density adjacent to the lucency.*

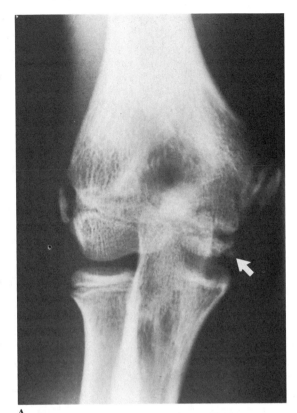

A

B

**Fig. 4-14.** *Fat-fluid level in tibial plateau fracture. A. The lateral view does not show the fracture. However, a fat-fluid level is seen in the suprapatellar bursa (arrows) caused by fat from the marrow cavity migrating into the disrupted joint space. This is seen only on a horizontal beam (cross-table) lateral film. The position allows the fat to float on top of the blood in the joint space. B. The AP view shows the slightly depressed fracture of the medial tibial plateau (arrow).*

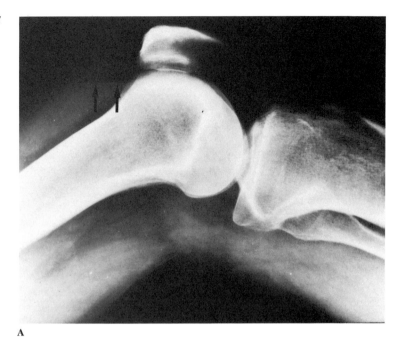

A

B

**Fig. 4-15.** *Paired fractures at opposite ends of long bones. The paired bones of the extremities may fracture at both ends. In this patient, there is a spiral fracture of the distal tibia. The lucency of the fracture is seen inferiorly (1), and the density caused by overlapping fragments is seen more proximally (2). The proximal fibula is also fractured (3). If a fracture occurs at one end of paired bones, the other end of these bones must be radiographed and examined carefully for a second injury.*

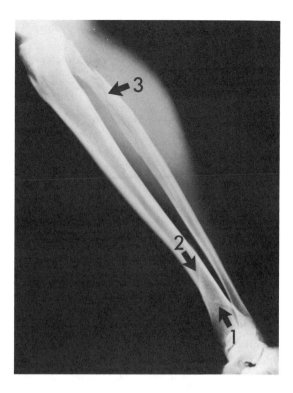

**b. Treatment.** Grades I and II generally are treated conservatively with a sling. Grade III separation frequently requires surgical correction.

2. **Effusion** (Fig. 4-17). Effusions may result from hemorrhage, infection, or trauma.

3. **Dislocation**

a. Anterior dislocation (Fig. 4-18)—humeral head resides in a subglenoid or subcoracoid position.

b. Posterior dislocation of the humeral head (Fig. 4-19)—more difficult to diagnose; usually caused by fall from height.

**Caveat.** AP view may look normal. A lateral view is mandatory.

**B. Elbow**

1. **Effusion** (Fig. 4-20). Abnormal position of fat pads is the key radiographic finding. The posterior fat pad normally is not seen.

2. **Dislocation** (Fig. 4-21). Frequently accompanies a fracture of the other forearm bone (e.g., radial fracture, ulnar dislocation). Dislocation may be difficult to detect. In a normal elbow, the axis of the radius should point to the capitellum.

3. **Radial head fracture** (see Fig. 4-6). This is often a subtle fracture. Joint hematoma may be the only finding. Multiple views may be necessary to detect the fracture itself.

**Fig. 4-16.** *Acromioclavicular separation. Films of both shoulders with and without the patient holding 5 pounds of weight should be obtained to assess the degree of separation. Weightbearing films are not needed if a film without weights shows separation greater than the width of the clavicle.* **A.** *Recognition of the injury depends on the demonstration of asymmetric **vertical** separation of the inferior margin of the acromion (1) from the inferior margin of the clavicle (2). Ligamentous injury has occurred on this patient's right side, where the acromion is displaced inferiorly from the clavicle by a distance greater than its width.* **B.** *On the left side, even with weights, there is no such vertical separation (arrows). The horizontal width of the acromioclavicular joint normally may appear greater on one side than the other because of a slight difference in the position of the patient.*

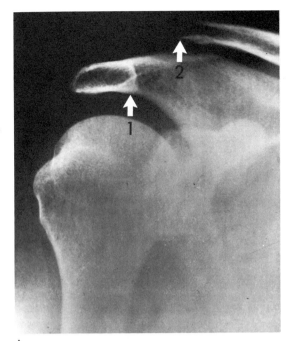

A

B

**Fig. 4-17.** *Shoulder effusion.*
*A. This patient with hemorrhagic bursitis demonstrates inferior displacement of the humeral head relative to the glenoid fossa.*
*B. Following aspiration of fluid from the joint, the normal relationship of the humeral head to the glenoid is restored. Such inferior subluxation is a nonspecific finding and may be seen if the patient has a hanging arm cast or a disease that has weakened the ligaments.*

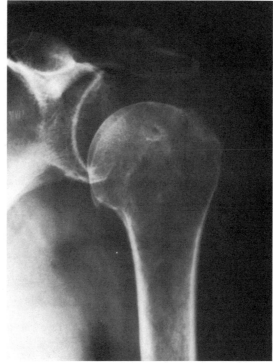

A

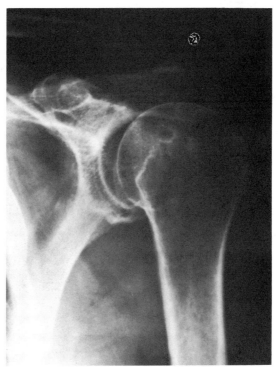

B

**Fig. 4-18.** *Anterior shoulder dislocation.* **A.** *The AP view shows an obvious dislocation, which is anterior. Posterior dislocations may not be visualized on the AP view. The humeral head typically moves inferiorly and medially in anterior dislocation.* **B.** *The Neer view (patient is rotated so the x-ray beam is tangential to the scapula) shows the anterior and inferior position of the humeral head relative to the glenoid. In a properly positioned Neer view, the glenoid (1) is in the center of a Y formed by the acromion (2), coracoid process (3), and body of the scapula (4). A normal humeral head will be centered over the glenoid (1). This is the best lateral view to check for dislocation.*

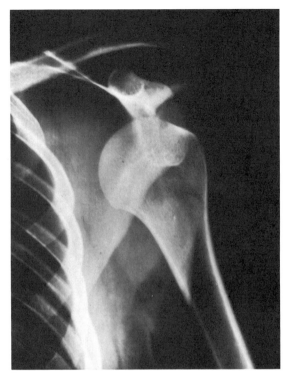

A

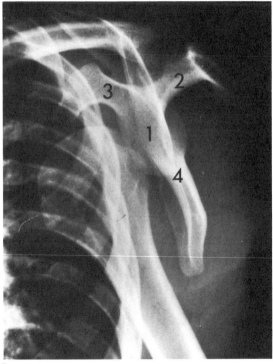

B

**Fig. 4-18** (*continued*). *C. In this transthoracic lateral view in a different patient, the shoulder is seen through the chest. The inferior aspect of the glenoid (**1**) is level with the middle of the humeral head, indicating inferior displacement of the head. This point of the glenoid fossa (**1**) should align with the surgical neck of the humerous (**2**), forming a continuous smooth curve. **D.** Another patient who had reduction of an anterior dislocation demonstrates a Hills-Sachs deformity (arrows), that is, a compression fracture of the humeral head where it impinges on the glenoid. Hills-Sachs deformity is seen in patients with chronic, repeated dislocations.*

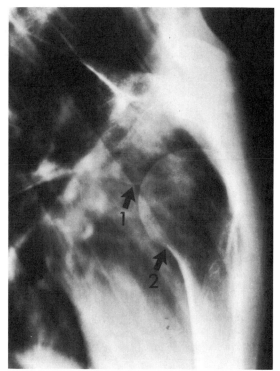

C

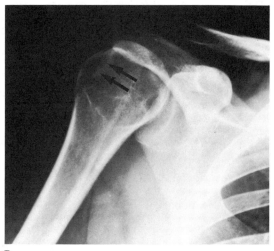

D

**Fig. 4-19.** *Posterior shoulder dislocation.* **A.** *Because the AP view may appear virtually normal, it is essential to obtain a lateral view (preferably a Neer or transaxial view). A clue on AP views is that the patient is not able to rotate the shoulder internally; thus, the humeral head consistently appears externally rotated. The margins of the greater and lesser tuberosities are seen laterally, as in this patient (arrows), in whom the humerus is externally rotated.* **B.** *The transaxillary lateral view is obtained by abducting the arm and shooting the x-ray beam through the axilla. This shows the posterior dislocation of the humeral head (1) relative to the glenoid (2). A compression fracture of the cortex of the humeral head is present (3). The anteriormost structures in this view are the coracoid process (4), the clavicle (5), and the acromion (6).*

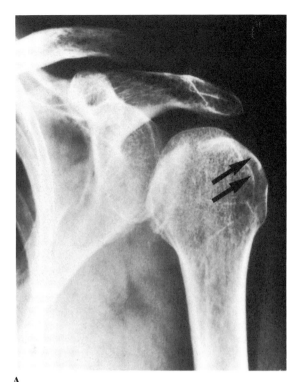

A

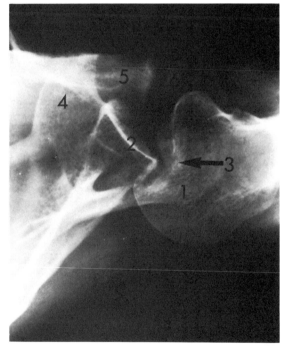

B

**Fig. 4-20.** *Elbow effusion. Elbow effusion is diagnosed by visualization of the posterior fat pad (1), which normally is in the olecranon fossa of the humerus and not visible. The anterior fat pad is barely seen normally, but in the presence of effusion becomes elevated and somewhat sail-shaped (2). If there has been trauma, an elbow effusion in adults implies a radial head fracture even if the fracture is not seen. Incidentally noted is a bone island in the radial head (3).*

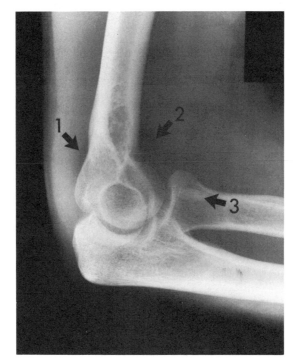

**Fig. 4-21.** *Fracture-dislocation of the elbow (Monteggia fracture). In this patient, the ulna is fractured while the radius has dislocated from the capitellum. Compare with the normal alignment demonstrated in Fig. 4-20.*

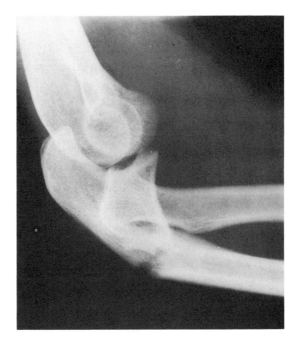

## C. Wrist

1. **Dislocations** (Figs. 4-22 and 4-23). Various dislocations may occur. If there is deformity of the wrist, a comparison view of the normal side is helpful in recognizing the dislocation.

2. **Fractures** (see Figs. 4-4, 4-5, and 4-7). Carpal bone fractures are difficult to detect, and careful scrutiny of each carpal bone is required in each view. The Colles' fracture is the most frequent fracture about the wrist. If a navicular fracture is suspected because of tenderness in the "snuffbox," special views of the navicular bone should be obtained. Navicular fractures may not be visible on the initial films; follow-up films in a week are indicated for persistent pain and frequently will demonstrate the fracture.

3. **Aseptic necrosis of navicular.** Failure to immobilize a navicular fracture leads to high likelihood of aseptic necrosis of the proximal portion of the navicular bone (Fig. 4-24).

## D. Knee

1. **Effusion** (Fig. 4-25). Visualization of the distended suprapatellar bursa is the clue to diagnosis.

2. **Dislocations**
   a. Patella (Fig. 4-26).
   b. Proximal fibula (Fig. 4-27).
   **Caveat.** AP view may look normal. Lateral view is mandatory.

3. **Fractures**
   a. **Tibial plateau** (Figs. 4-14 and 4-28). These may be avulsions of the tibial spines or fractures resulting from compression of the tibial plateau. Oblique views of the knee may be especially helpful in demonstrating plateau fractures. A fat-fluid level seen in the suprapatellar bursa implies a fracture until proved otherwise.
   b. **Patella** (Fig. 4-29). A patellar fracture that is horizontal will be best seen on the lateral view. However, patellar fractures are frequently vertical and may be seen only on a skyline view. **If patellar fracture is suspected, the skyline view may uniquely display the fracture.**

4. **Bipartite patella** (see Fig. 4-12). This normal variant should not be confused with a fracture. Its characteristic features include smooth edges, presence of circumferential cortical bone, and location in the upper outer quadrant of the patella.

## E. Ankle and foot

1. **Ankle effusion** (Fig. 4-30). As in elbow and knee effusions, the distended bursa is the radiographic finding.

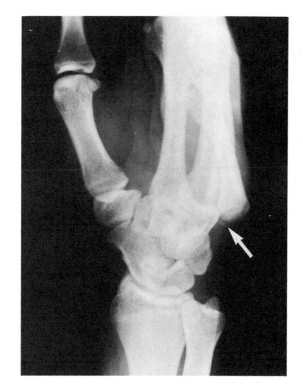

**Fig. 4-22.** *Metacarpal dislocation. There is dislocation of the fourth and fifth metacarpals as well as a small avulsion fracture (arrow). Comparison with the normal side is helpful in diagnosing dislocations.*

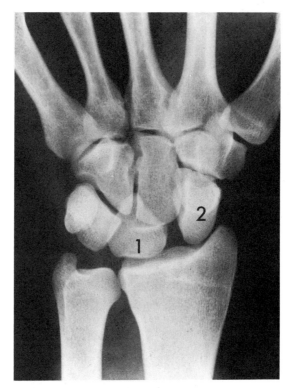

**Fig. 4-23.** *Lunate dislocation. The lunate (1) has assumed a pie-shaped or triangular configuration on this posteroanterior (PA) view. This is characteristic of anterior dislocation of the lunate. Also note the distance between the navicular (2) and lunate bones is widened. Compare these findings with the normal quadrilateral or rectangular appearance of the lunate seen in Fig. 4-5.*

**Fig. 4-24.** *Aseptic necrosis following a navicular fracture. Aseptic necrosis involves the proximal part of the navicular bone (1), which is deprived of its blood supply by the fracture (2). The finding that indicates aseptic necrosis is increased density of the proximal part of the navicular bone compared with adjacent carpal bones (e.g., lunate [3] or capitate [4]). Comparison with the density of the distal part of the navicular (5) is not reliable because the distal part of the navicular bone may appeaar more dense normally in this projection owing to its oblique orientation.*

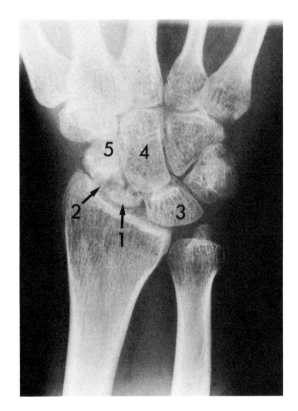

**Fig. 4-25.** *Knee effusion. The presence of knee effusion is determined by measuring the horizontal distance between the suprapatellar fat, which is triangular (1), and the prefemoral fat (2). Normally this distance measures 2 to 4 mm. A distance greater than 5 mm implies an effusion. Occasionally the superior margin of the bursa is seen (3).*

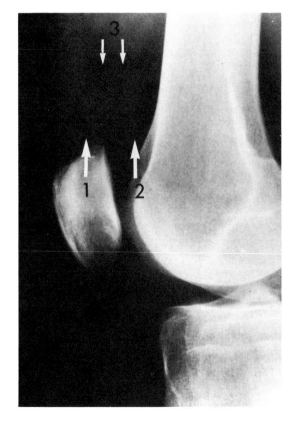

**Fig.** 4-26. *Patellar dislocation. Comparison of A (dislocated) and B (reduced) demonstrates the lateral displacement of the patella. Note that there is little difference in projection between these two views; the amount of overlap of the tibia and fibula is about the same. The patella may also dislocate superiorly if the infrapatellar ligament is torn.*

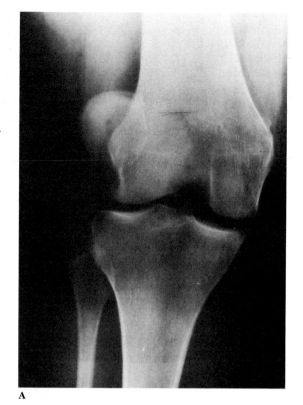

A

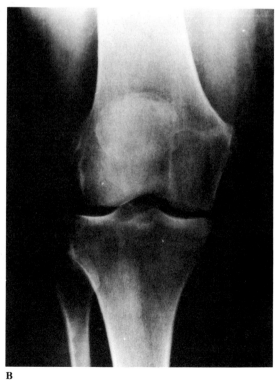

B

**Fig. 4-27.** *Dislocation of proximal fibula.* **A.** *This dislocation is subtle and easily missed. The AP view shows that the right fibula (1) is a little more lateral than is the left fibula (2). The position of the patella relative to the tibia indicates very little difference in rotation of the two knees.* **B.** *The lateral view shows the fibula (1) to be anterior to its normal position of articulation with the tibia, identified by the faintly seen line of increased density in the tibia (2). Fig. 4-14A shows the normal relationship in the lateral projection.*

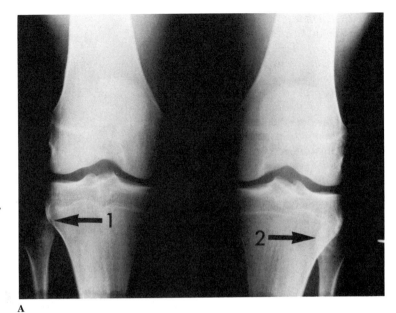

A

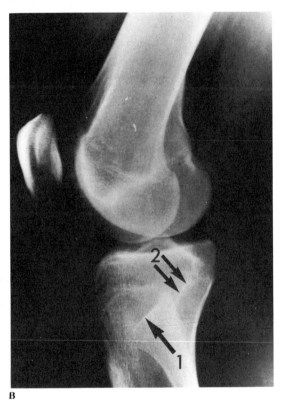

B

**Fig. 4-28.** *Avulsion of anterior tibial spine. Avulsion of the tibial spine occurs with excessive stress on the cruciate ligaments. Such a lesion may be overlooked or mistaken for a loose body.* **A.** *On the AP view, the avulsion is barely visible (arrows).* **B.** *The lateral view leaves no doubt that the fragment is an avulsion because of the lack of cortex at the anterior and inferior aspects of the fragment (arrows).*

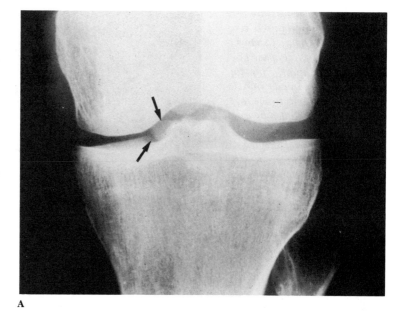

A

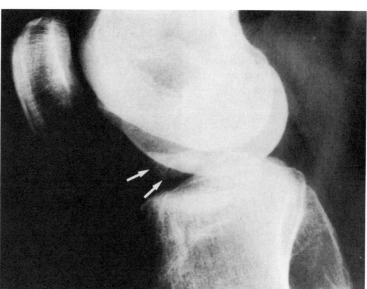

B

**Fig. 4-29.** *Patellar fracture. There is no doubt that this is a fracture. The fracture lucency is at the medial aspect of the patella, whereas bipartite patella occurs laterally. In addition, the trabeculae adjacent to the lucency are not bounded by any cortical bone. This view is a "skyline" view, in which the knee is flexed and the x-ray beam is directed parallel to the patellofemoral joint.*

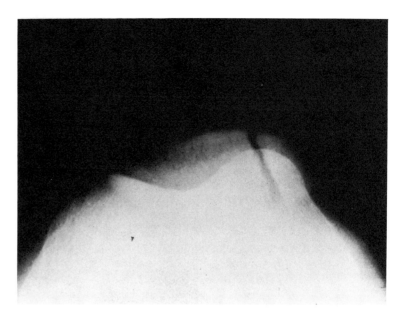

**Fig. 4-30.** *Ankle effusion. An ankle effusion is seen only in the lateral view. The fluid in the joint space is outlined by the fat anterior and posterior to the tibiotalar joint (arrows).*

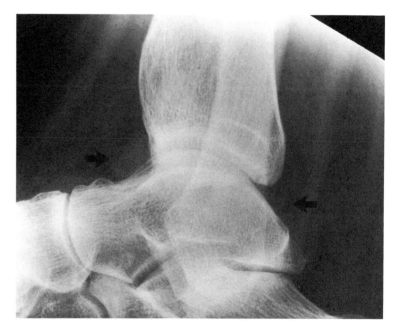

2. **Ligamentous injury** (Fig. 4-31). Views in inversion or eversion with stress on the ankle joint may be required. If no fracture is seen but significant injury is suspected clinically, stress views may help document the extent of ligamentous injury.

3. **Dislocations** (Fig. 4-32). Dislocations may be subtle. Comparison with the noninjured side may be essential.

4. **Fractures**

   a. **Stress fracture** (Fig. 4-33). A stress (march) fracture may be invisible or barely visible initially. Follow-up examination in 1 to 2 weeks shows periosteal reaction resulting from the fracture. Follow-up examination is indicated when no fracture is seen initially but symptoms persist.

   b. **Lisfranc fracture** (Fig. 4-34). Easily overlooked, these fractures of the proximal metatarsals should be searched for meticulously. They may occur with or without dislocation of the metatarsals. Their incidence is increased in diabetics.

   c. **Axial fractures** (Figs. 4-35 and 4-36). Fractures may occur parallel to the axis of the bone as opposed to the more usual transverse fracture. Tarsal fractures may be difficult to see because of the overlap of the tarsal bones on the radiographs; various films in different degrees of obliquity may demonstrate the fractures.

   d. **Calcaneus fracture** (Fig. 4-37). In addition to comparison views with the opposite side, a tangential view of the heel (Harris view) may be helpful. Flattening of the Boehler's angle of the calcaneus suggests a fracture, even if the fracture line itself is not seen.

   e. **Fracture of proximal fifth metatarsal** (Jones fracture) versus unfused epiphysis (Fig. 4-38). Lack of fusion of the epiphysis of the fifth metatarsal is easily confused with a fracture. A proximal fifth metatarsal fracture may occur in association with ankle injuries. The fracture often will be visible on the edge of the ankle radiograph—a classic "corner of the film fracture."

III. **Osteomyelitis.** Osteomyelitis presently is uncommon, due in part to potent and specific antibiotics. It is seen more frequently in children than in adults. In the pediatric population, it commonly is caused by a remote source of infection that spread hematogenously. In adults, the source is usually more obvious. Chronic infections in the feet of diabetics; penetrating injuries with sharp, dirty objects; and open compound fractures are settings for osteomyelitis.

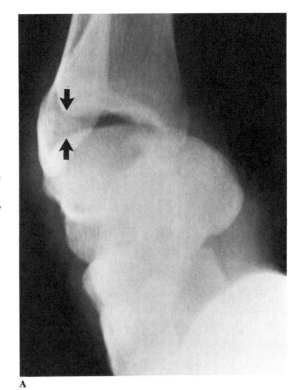

**Fig. 4-31.** *Importance of stress views to demonstrate ligamentous injury. Comparison of the right tibiotalar joint in* **A** *(tear) and* **B** *(normal left side) demonstrates asymmetric widening of the joint laterally on the patient's right side where the calcaneofibular and talocalcaneal ligaments have been torn (arrows). Both views were obtained while inversion stress was placed on the ankle. Physical examination must provide the clue to injury; in the absence of avulsion fractures, x-rays may appear normal without stress and stress views.*

A

B

**Fig. 4-32.** *Metatarsal disloca-tion.* **A.** *The proximal second metatarsal (arrow) is fractured and there is lateral dislocation of the second through fifth meta-tarsals.* **B.** *Comparison with the normal side facilitates recogni-tion of the dislocation. (The pic-ture of the normal side has been reversed for ease of comparison.) Note the difference from* **A** *in the relationship of the fifth metatar-sal and the cuboid (arrow).*

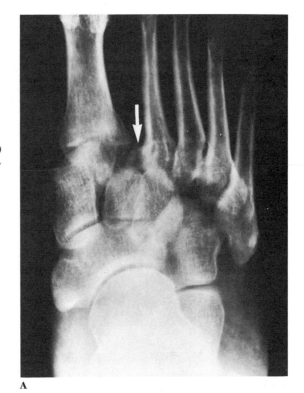

A

B

**Fig. 4-33.** *Stress fracture may not be seen on initial x-rays.* **A.** *The patient complained of metatarsal pain after jogging. These films failed to demonstrate a fracture.* **B.** *Twelve days later, a repeat examination shows periosteal reaction (arrows), the hallmark of a healing stress fracture.*

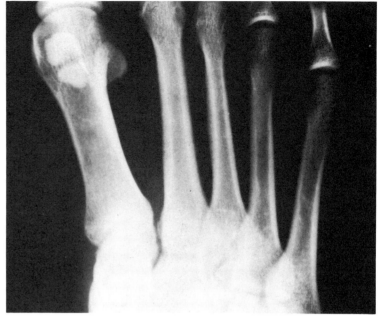

A

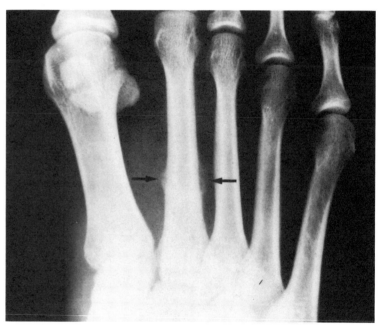

B

**Fig. 4-34.** *Fracture of proximal metatarsals (arrows). This is called the Lisfranc fracture and may occur with or without dislocation. It is an easy fracture to overlook unless specifically searched for. It is seen more frequently in diabetic patients.*

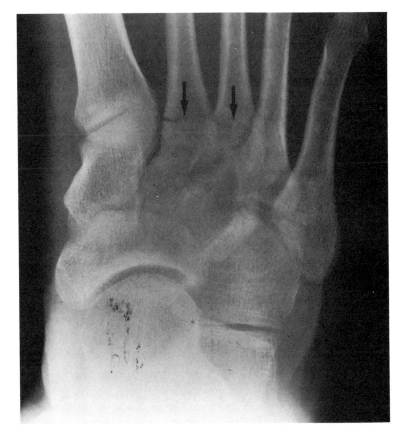

**Fig. 4-35.** *Axial orientation of tibial fracture. The AP (A) and lateral (B) views demonstrate an obvious fracture running almost parallel to the axis of the tibia. Such a fracture results when the force of injury is transmitted parallel to the axis of the bone. Not so easily seen is the fracture of the posterior malleolus. The cortical disruption is indicated by the arrow.*

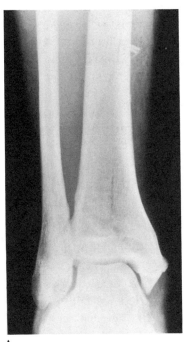

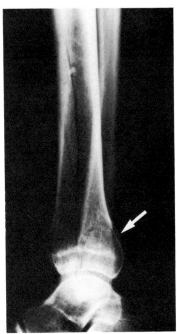

A                                              B

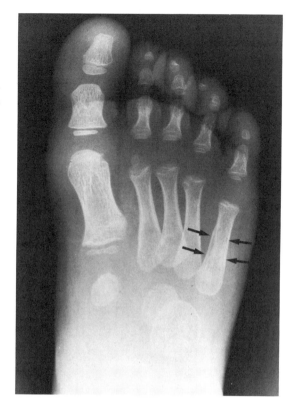

**Fig. 4-36.** *Axial orientation of metatarsal fracture. This fracture is different from the usual transverse fracture. No cortical break is seen. The only findings are the lucencies running almost parallel to the bony cortex in the fifth metatarsal (arrows).*

*Staphylococcus aureus* is the most common organism causing osteomyelitis. Gram-negative organisms are next most frequent. *Salmonella* osteomyelitis occurs in patients with sickle cell disease.

Osteomyelitis may be acute or chronic or it may cause bone abscess (Brodie's abscess). A final uncommon variant is sclerosing osteomyelitis.

**A. Radiographic findings** (Figs. 4-39 and 4-40)

  **1. Soft tissue.** The earliest x-ray findings of osteomyelitis are in the soft tissues.

    **a.** Swelling

    **b.** Disruption of normal fat planes, especially those adjacent to the bone

  **2. Osseous.** These manifestations may be delayed 7 to 10 days on x-rays.

    **a.** Patchy lucency of bone often is the initial manifestation.

    **b.** Periostitis.

    **c.** Metaphysis is most frequently affected.

    **d.** Frank bony destruction and moth-eaten appearance are late findings.

  **3.** Chronic osteomyelitis findings

    **a. Sequestra**—dead isolated pieces of bone

**Fig. 4-37.** *Calcaneus fracture results in flat Boehler's angle.* **A.** *The Harris view (AP projection of the posterior part of the calcaneus) reveals the linear lucencies of a comminuted fracture (arrows).* **B.** *The lateral view demonstrates a cortical break (white arrow) and the fracture lucency (straight black arrows). In addition, Boehler's angle has been flattened (curved black arrow). Boehler's angle is formed by the intersection of two lines drawn from the superiormost part of the posterior and middle portion of the calcaneus and the middle and anterior portion of the calcaneus. This angle is normally 20 to 40 degrees. Decrease in this angle may be the only sign of fracture.*

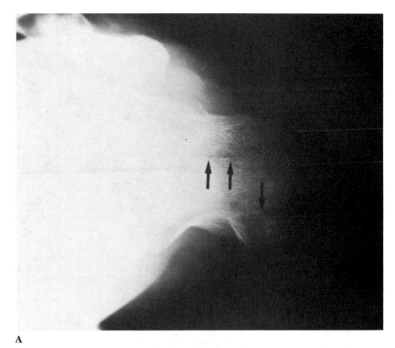

A

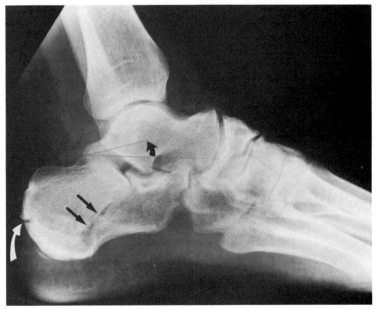

B

**Fig. 4-38.** *Fifth metatarsal epiphysis versus fracture.* **A.** *The unfused epiphysis may persist into adult life. Note that its orientation is parallel to the axis of the fifth metatarsal and its edges are smoothly rounded. Comparison with the opposite side may be helpful.* **B.** *Fractures of the proximal fifth metatarsal are almost always transverse in orientation, the edges are not smooth, and acute angles always suggest fracture (arrow).*

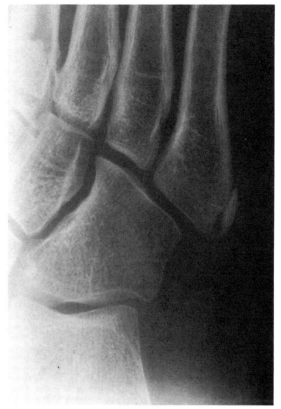

A

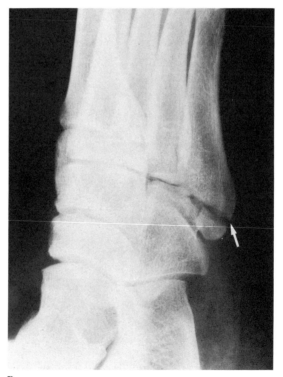

B

**Fig. 4-39.** *Osteomyelitis involves the second through fifth toes. With gas in the soft tissues, lytic bone destruction may be difficult to discern. Note the cortical destruction of the distal fourth metacarpal (arrows) in comparison with the normal second. The phalanges of the fourth toe are almost completely destroyed.*

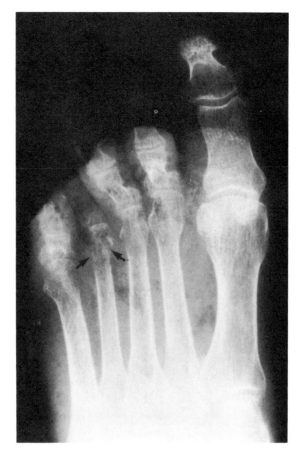

**Fig. 4-40.** *Staphylococcal osteomyelitis has resulted in lytic destruction of the proximal tibia.*

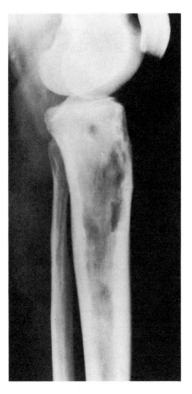

**b. Involucra**—heavy dense bone built from periosteal new bone around the original shaft

4. Radionuclide bone scanning or other agents with an affinity for inflammation have become helpful in the diagnosis.

**IV. Arthritis.** The arthritides encompass a vast spectrum of diseases, which frequently present with systemic manifestations. Specific serologic, bacteriologic, and synovioanalytic studies are diagnostic but not always immediately available. Radiographic patterns of arthritides offer clues to the diagnosis. This section will highlight only those arthritides relevant in the emergency room setting.

**A. Pyogenic (septic) arthritis** (Fig. 4-41)

1. This is perhaps the most important diagnosis to make or strongly consider in the emergency room because of its potential for rapid bone destruction and dissemination throughout the body.

2. Clinical clues usually are helpful and may help point to gonococcal (venereal or pharyngeal lesions), staphylococcal (adjacent osteomyelitis or injury), gram-negative, or mixed infection.

3. Early radiographic findings
   **a.** Soft tissue swelling
   **b.** Joint effusion
   **c.** Usually monarticular

4. Osseous findings
   **a.** Erosion of articular cartilage with resultant narrowing of the joint space is seen.
   **b.** Later destruction of the joint takes place.
   **c.** These findings generally occur on **both** sides of the joint.
   **d.** Bony density often remains intact, especially if the process is virulent.

**B. Gouty arthritis** (Fig. 4-42)

1. A differential diagnosis of pyogenic arthritis due to fever, localized warmth, tenderness, and swelling of the affected joint.

2. May affect more than one joint; most frequently first metatarsophalangeal joint (podagra).

3. Occurs with a 9:1 male preponderance.

4. Urate arthropathy may also occur in patients taking chemotherapeutic drugs or diuretics due to hyperuricosuria.

5. Radiographic findings
   **a.** Soft tissue swelling and joint effusion are earlier findings
   **b.** Calcified (or noncalcified) soft tissue masses (tophi).
   **c.** Localized, circumscribed bony lucency
   **d.** Later, juxta-articular erosions

**Fig. 4-41.** *Staphylococcal arthritis involved the knee joint in this 62-year-old patient.* **A.** *There is a joint effusion (straight arrows). The joint space is slightly narrowed on the AP view (**B**), implying erosion of cartilage. The bony cortex is eroded (curved arrows).*

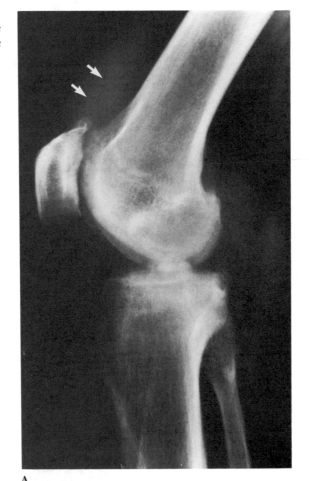

A

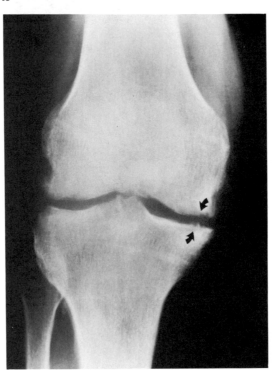

B

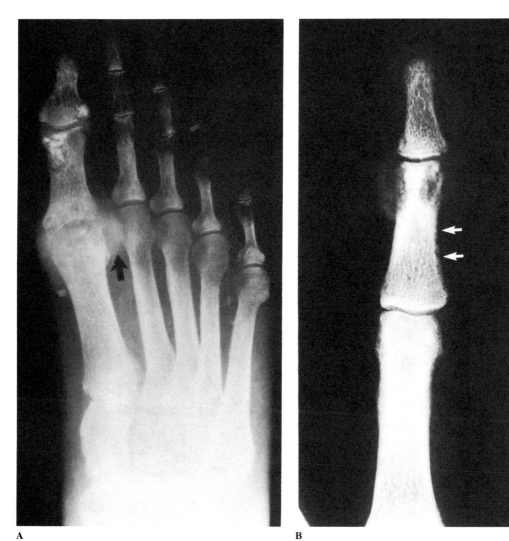

**A**

**B**

**Fig. 4-42.** *Gout involving the great toe (podagra) (A) demonstrates the dense tophi (arrow) as well as juxta-articular and articular erosions. Similar findings are seen at the distal interphalangeal joint of the finger in the same patient (B). Of note is the subperiosteal resorption of bone (arrows), which results from hyperparathyroidism secondary to gout-induced nephropathy.*

**Fig. 4-43.** *Rheumatoid arthritis results in cartilage destruction, bony erosions, and ulnar deviation of the fifth metacarpophalangeal joint. The "pencil in cup" bone and joint appearance is a characteristic noted (straight arrow). The proximal joints including the carpus are more severely involved (curved arrow).*

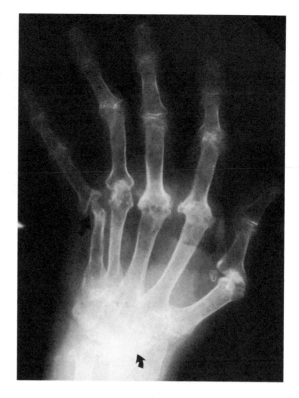

**C. Rheumatoid arthritis and variants** (Fig. 4-43)

1. Not commonly seen acutely in adults in the emergency room setting.
2. Juvenile rheumatoid arthritis may be seen as a systemic illness at the emergency room
3. Radiographic findings
   **a.** Earliest
      **(1)** Soft tissue swelling
      **(2)** Characteristically **symmetric**
      **(3)** Proximal interphalangeal and metacarpophalangeal joints, knees, and ankles involved
   **b.** Early osseous findings
      **(1)** Juxta-articular osteoporosis
      **(2)** Marginal joint erosions
   **c. Late findings** include loss of joint space, subluxation, and symmetric multiplicity of joint involvement.

**D. Sacroiliitis and ankylosing spondylitis:**

1. May occur as an independent disease or in association with another disease (e.g., with inflammatory bowel disease).
2. Limited either to sacroiliac joints or may ascend in the spine.
3. Sacroiliac joint disease shows wide joint space from effusion initially.

**Fig. 4-44.** *Psoriatic arthritis results in destruction of the fifth distal interphalangeal (DIP) joint (white arrow). Erosions are also seen at the carpometacarpal joint of the thumb (black arrow). The soft-tissue and bony changes are similar to those of rheumatoid arthritis. Asymmetric involvement, especially of the DIP joints, is characteristic of psoriatic arthritis and differentiates it from rheumatoid arthritis.*

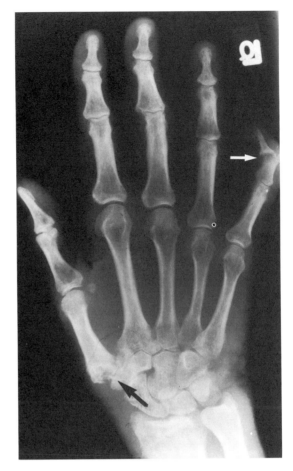

4. Sacroiliac joints narrow and become sclerotic later.
5. Advanced disease involves spinal ankylosis with ligamentous calcification (see Fig. 3-23).

E. **Psoriatic arthritis** (Fig. 4-44)
1. May present **before** characteristic skin and nail changes (10–15 percent of instances)
2. Distal interphalangeal joints affected frequently and nonsymmetrically
3. Multiple joints often involved
4. May involve sacroiliac joints

F. **Osteoarthritis (degenerative joint disease)** (Fig. 4-45)
1. Common after bony trauma or in the elderly.
2. Usually a chronic problem and frequently observed on emergency room radiographs, but usually **not** acute.
3. Radiographic findings
   a. No specific acute findings, since it is a chronic process.
   b. Bony changes including spurring, sclerosis and cystic degeneration of joints, and loss of joint space.

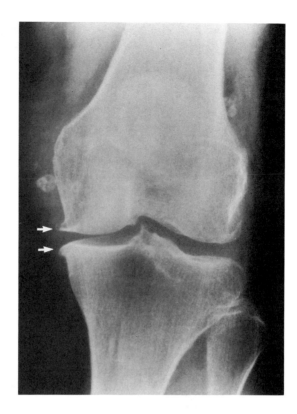

**Fig. 4-45.** *Osteoarthritis is characterized by spur formation as an early finding (arrows).*

4. Weight bearing (or traumatized) bones most frequently affected, e.g., hips, spine, knees (see Figs. 2-16 and 3-17).

G. **Hemophiliac arthropathy** (Fig. 4-46)

  1. In hemophiliacs, bleeding into joints may be a cause for recurrent emergency room visits.

  2. Knees are involved most frequently.

  3. Radiographic findings

     a. Joint effusion.

     b. Loss of joint space because of cartilage destruction.

     c. Ends of affected bones may enlarge because of disproportionate growth from hypervascularity.

V. **Soft tissue problems**

A. **Periarticular disease**

  1. Includes bursitis, tendinitis, fibrosis

  2. Frequent cause for emergency room visits owing to pain and limited range of motion

  3. Shoulder often involved

  4. Radiographic findings

     a. Soft tissue calcification juxtaposed to the joint; calcification seen in only 30 to 50 percent of instances; conversely, asymptomatic calcifications frequently are seen (Fig. 4-47).

**Fig. 4-46.** *Hemophilia has resulted in minimal erosions of the medial joint margin. There are juxta-articular erosions, which are thought to result from intraosseous hemorrhage (arrow).*

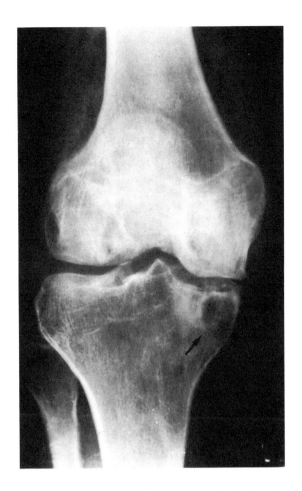

**Fig. 4-47.** *Calcifications in the shoulder bursa are seen adjacent to the intertubercular groove (arrow).*

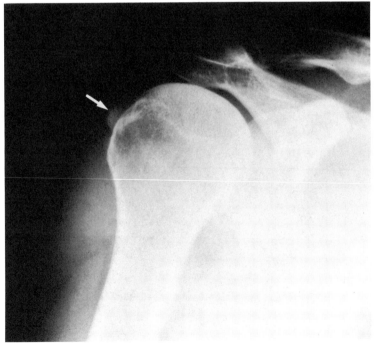

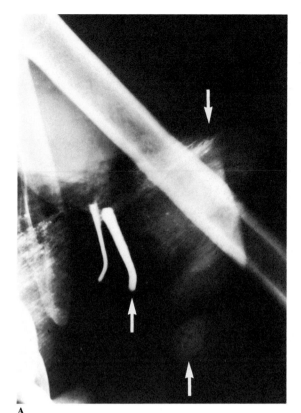

A

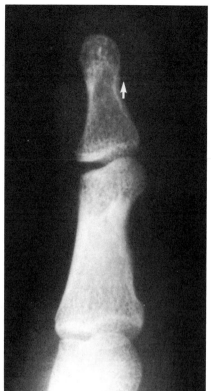

B

**Fig. 4-48.** *In patient **A**, a large piece of wood penetrated the axilla. The difference in density is apparent among the wood, extraneous metallic objects, and plastic button (arrows). In patient **B**, a small sliver of glass penetrated the finger (arrow). To be certain a foreign body is within, rather than overlying, the soft tissues, two views 90 degrees apart must demonstrate the object. If uncertainty persists, fluoroscopy may be used for localization.*

**b.** Patchy osteoporosis seen if immobilization has occurred because of pain.

**B. Foreign body** (Fig. 4-48)

1. Common indication for x-ray with penetrating trauma or injury that has disrupted skin.
2. Metal, glass, and thick wood all visible.
3. Radiographic findings
   **a.** May not be visualized on only one projection.
   **b.** Need 90-degree tangential views.
   **c.** Physician should check for adjacent osseous disruption.
4. Xeroradiography very helpful for foreign body films.
5. Radiographic needle localization may be necessary for removal of the foreign body.

SELECTED READINGS

Abbitt PL, Riddervold HO. Carpal tunnel view: Helpful adjuvant for unrecognized fractures of the carpus. Skeletal Radiol 16:45, 1987.

Abel MS. Jogger's fracture and other stress fractures of the lumbosacral spine. Skeletal Radiol 13:221, 1985.

Altman R, Asch E, Bloch D, et al. Development of criteria for the classification and reporting of osteoarthritis: Classification of osteoarthritis of the knee. Arthritis Rheum 29:1039, 1986.

Giachino AA, Hammon DI. The relationship between oblique fractures of medial malleolus and concomitant fractures of the anterolateral aspect of the tibial plafond. J Bone Joint Surg 69A:381, 1987.

Hall-Craggs MA, Shorvon PJ, Chapman M. Assessment of the radial head–capitellum view and the dorsal fat-pad sign in acute elbow trauma. AJR 145:607, 1985.

Lawson JR. Symptomatic radiographic variants in extremities. Radiology 157:625, 1985.

Page AC. Critical evaluation of the radial head–capitellum view in elbow trauma. AJR 146:81, 1986.

Ruby LK, Stinson J, Belsky MR. The natural history of scaphoid nonunion. J Bone Joint Surg 67A:728, 1985.

Singer AM, Naimark A, Felson D, et al. Comparison of overhead and cross-table lateral views for detection of knee-joint effusion. AJR 144:973, 1985.

Tehranzadeh J. Spectrum of avulsion and avulsion-like injuries of the musculoskeletal system. Radiographics 7:945, 1987.

Williamson SL, Seibert JJ, Glasier CM, et al. Complications of fractures elucidated by bone scans. Clin Nucl Med 12:260, 1987.

Yeager BA, Dalinka MK. Radiology of trauma to the wrist: Dislocations, fracture dislocations and instability patterns. Skeletal Radiol 13:120, 1985.

Zlatkin MB, Bjorkengren A, Sartoris DJ, et al. Stress fractures of distal tibia and calcaneus subsequent to acute fractures of the tibia and fibula. AJR 149:329, 1987.

# 5 The Chest

*Paul Stark, Eric vanSonnenberg, and James T. Rhea*

Up to 40 percent of emergency room films are chest x-rays. The frequency of use of these studies reflects their importance in triage and management of emergency room patients. Correct interpretation of chest x-rays helps determine the cause and therapy of many true emergencies. A systematic approach to the study and interpretation of the chest x-ray is presented in the first part of this chapter. The second part describes specific thoracic abnormalities and diseases.

Chest x-ray reading is as much an art as any aspect of radiology. Recognition of fine distinctions and subtle clues is necessary for correct interpretation. Thus, correctly interpreted chest x-rays can differentiate intrinsic pulmonary disease from that secondary to cardiac disease, can distinguish mediastinal from hilar disease, permits diagnosis of nodules and pneumothorax and differentiates artifacts, and allows apt estimates of cardiac size, which helps categorize dyspnea problems. As with other x-ray studies, abnormalities are obscured by poor technique; thus repeat films are mandatory, lest important observations be missed.

SYSTEMATIC VIEWING
METHOD

I. **Lungs and pleura** ( Fig. 5-1 )
   A. Comparing the lungs from side to side helps discern asymmetry.
      1. Increased density—indicates pneumonia, tumor, bleeding, fluid of any type. Rotation ( Fig. 5-2 ) and overlying soft tissue ( Fig. 5-3 ) may simulate disease.
      2. Decreased density—bullae, pneumothorax (see Fig. 7-4 ), hypoperfusion, rotation
   B. Particularly difficult portions of the lung in which abnormalities may be overlooked include:
      1. **Lung apices,** where the clavicle, first rib, and costal cartilage overlie the lung
      2. **Lung bases**—abdominal films often permit better visualization of the lung bases than chest x-ray in the anteroposterior ( AP ) projection.
      3. Perihilar regions, where the abnormalities may masquerade as vessels

**Fig. 5-1.** *These normal chest posteroanterior (PA) (A) and lateral (B) views should be compared with subsequent abnormal films. The lungs are symmetrically lucent, the patient has taken a deep inspiration (diaphragm is about at the tenth rib on the PA view); the borders of the heart, peripheral vessels, and hilar vessels are sharply defined; and the costophrenic angles are sharp and clear. The patient is a 24-year-old female, and slight rotation on the PA view results in compression of the left breast tissue but not the right, which appears as a rounded density projected over the right fifth anterior rib. Exposure of the film ideally allows easy visualization of peripheral vessels as well as the lucency of the trachea and main stem bronchi through the mediastinum and the branching vessels through the heart.*

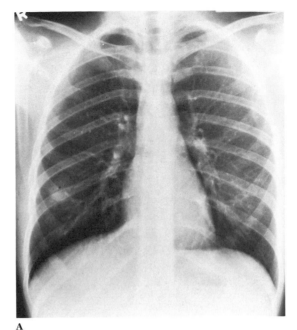

A

B

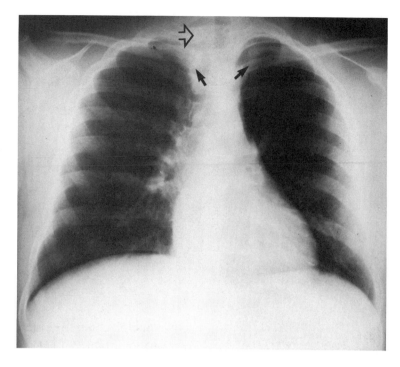

**Fig. 5-2.** *Rotation causes the lungs to appear asymmetrically lucent. This is considered a normal variation, since the lungs become obliquely positioned in the thorax. In this patient the left lung appears more lucent than the right. The amount of rotation can be ascertained by comparing an anterior structure such as the end of the clavicle (solid arrows) with a posterior structure such as the spinous process (open arrow). In a straight film the spinous process would project in the midline between the clavicular heads. Note that this slight right anterior oblique positioning also makes the right hilum more prominent than the left.*

    **4.** Areas overlying the vertebrae on lateral or posteroanterior (PA) radiographs

    **5.** Retrocardiac area

  **C.** **Pleural sulci** should be checked on both frontal and lateral projections for small amounts of fluid.

  **D.** **Lung volumes** should be assessed

    **1.** **Small volumes** (Fig. 5-4) are associated with

      **a.** Poor inspiratory effort or true small volumes.

      **b.** Vessel crowding and indistinctness at the lung bases—this spurious appearance of indistinct vessels may be confused with interstitial pulmonary edema.

      **c.** True small volumes indicate restrictive lung disease.

    **2.** Large lung volumes

      **a.** May indicate obstructive lung disease (chronic or acute, such as asthma).

      **b.** In large people, they are normal.

  **E.** **Diaphragmatic surfaces** should be checked for the following (smooth undulations are a normal variant):

    **1.** Position (usually equal level or right side slightly higher than left)

    **2.** Calcification

    **3.** Subpulmonic pleural effusion

**II.** **Heart** (see Fig. 5-1)

  **A.** The normal heart should traverse less than half the transverse distance from inner rib to inner rib at the level of the diaphragm if the patient has taken a full inspiration.

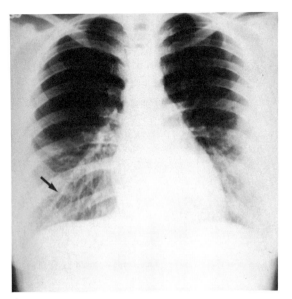

**A**

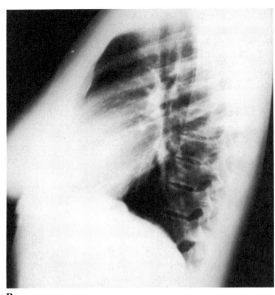

**B**

**Fig. 5-3.** *Overlying breast tissue makes the lower lungs appear more dense than the upper on the PA view ( A ). The sharp definition of the heart borders and lower vessels ( e.g., arrow ) suggest that increased density is not consolidation. B. The normal lateral view confirms the absence of consolidation in the lower lungs. In the normal lateral projection, the lower thoracic vertebrae become more lucent with caudal progression.*

B. **Specific chamber enlargement** often adds etiologic information ( Table 5-1 ) ( Figs. 5-5 and 5-6 ).

C. Large lung volumes ( chronic obstructive pulmonary disease [COPD] ) may cause the heart to appear relatively small and underestimate true heart size.

D. **Pericardial effusion** is most reliably diagnosed ( by plain film ) on the lateral view ( Fig. 5-7 ).

III. **Hila and vasculature** ( see Fig. 5-1 )

A. The hila should be **smooth** and relatively **symmetric.**

B. Presence of lumpy or **asymmetric** hila generally indicates adenopathy ( Fig. 5-8 ).

C. The left hilum is almost always higher than the right. Abnormal hilar position may be the sole indicator of lobar collapse.

D. **Vessels** should gradually taper as they branch **peripherally** from the hila.

E. Smooth hilar enlargement with abrupt vessel tapering characterizes pulmonary arterial hypertension ( see Fig. 5-6 ).

IV. **Mediastinum** ( see Fig. 5-1 )

A. Mediastinal contours are normally smooth and without masslike borders.

B. Thymic tissue is visualized routinely in infants and may be seen as late as age 12 on chest x-ray. In adults, excess tissue in the area of the thymus suggests tumor ( Fig. 5-9 ).

C. With symptoms and signs of acute or subacute **upper airway** disease, the trachea and main bronchi should be checked carefully for obstructing lesions ( Fig. 5-10 ).

D. The aorta becomes tortuous with age, as does the innomi-

**Fig. 5-4.** *The problems of poor inspiration. Subtle abnormalities may be missed, and there may be a false impression of consolidation, congestive heart failure, and cardiomegaly. Sequential expiration (**A**) and inspiration (**B**) films in this normal patient demonstrate the marked effects of a "poor inspiration": added density, fuzzy cardiac and vascular borders, and a false appearance of cardiomegaly.*

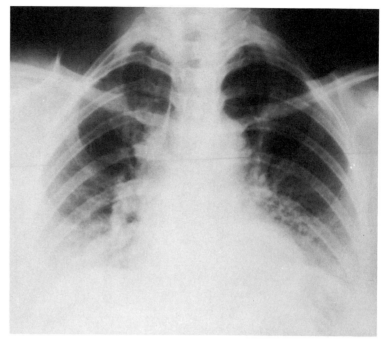

A

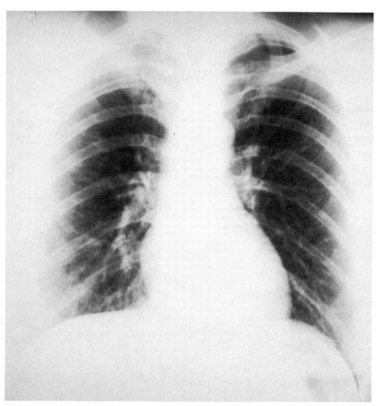

B

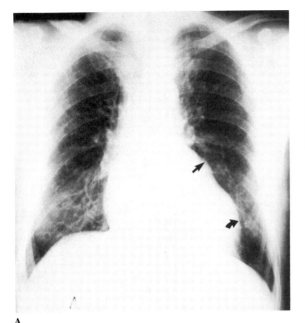

A

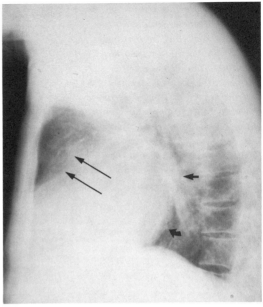

B

**Fig. 5-5.** *Left atrial and left ventricular enlargement are seen in this patient with both mitral stenosis and mitral insufficiency. Compare with Fig. 5-1 and note the appearance of the left atrial appendage on the PA (**A,** straight arrow) and the enlarged left atrium on the lateral (**B,** short straight arrow). The left ventricle enlarges to the left and posteriorly (curved arrows). The retrosternal space remains clear with left atrial and ventricular enlargement (long straight arrows).*

**Table 5-1.** *Etiology of Specific Cardiac Chamber Enlargement*

| Enlarged chamber | Etiology |
| --- | --- |
| Left ventricle | Hypertension, aortic valvular or subvalvular stenosis |
| Left ventricle, left atrium | Arteriosclerotic heart disease, mitral insufficiency |
| Left atrium, right ventricle, right atrium | Mitral stenosis |
| Right atrium, right ventricle | Pulmonary outflow disease, primary pulmonary disease |
| Right atrium | Tricuspid valve disease |

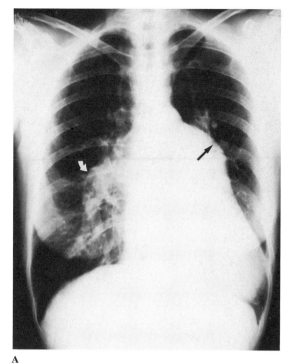

**A**

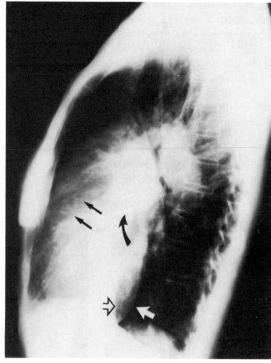

**B**

**Fig. 5-6.** *Posteroanterior (A) and lateral (B) views showing enlargement of the right ventricle, pulmonary outflow tract (A, straight arrow), and proximal pulmonary arteries (curved arrows) in this patient with pulmonary arterial hypertension. On the lateral film (B), the enlarged right pulmonary artery (curved arrow) is seen anterior to the lucency of the main stem bronchi. The rounded density slightly above and posterior is the enlarged left pulmonary artery. The large right ventricle has partially "filled in" the retrosternal space (paired straight arrows). This results in posterior displacement of the left ventricle (white straight arrow). The vertical line (open arrow) on the lateral view is the inferior vena cava.*

nate artery in the right paratracheal region (Fig. 5-11). The latter may be confused with a mass.

   **E. Mediastinal shift** may be caused by
     **1.** Volume loss (shift toward)
     **2.** Mass or large pleural fluid effect (shift away from)
     **3.** Bronchial obstruction from foreign body or tumor (shift away from)
     **4.** Tension pneumothorax (shift away from) (Fig. 5-12)
   **F.** Lucent accentuation of mediastinal structures indicates pneumomediastinum (Fig. 5-13).

**V. Bones**
   **A.** The major categories of osseous abnormalities likely to be noted on chest x-ray include:
     **1. Trauma**
     **2. Tumor**
     **3. Congenital conditions**
   **B.** In trauma and suspected metastatic disease, specific coned views of the area in question offer more detail than chest x-ray (see Fig. 7-8).
   **C.** Asymmetry is a reliable indicator of abnormality.
   **D. Caveat. If a bone abnormality is suspected, obtain bone films.** Chest radiograph technique is not intended for bones, and lesions may not be apparent.

**Fig. 5-7.** *Pericardial effusion may appear as ventricular enlargement on the posteroanterior view (**A**). The diagnosis is made on the lateral view (**B**), where a vertical band of fluid density is seen to separate the epicardial and pericardial fat just anterior to the heart (arrows). The patient also has a pleural effusion. Note the increased density posteriorly on the lateral view filling in one of these posterior costophrenic sulci.*

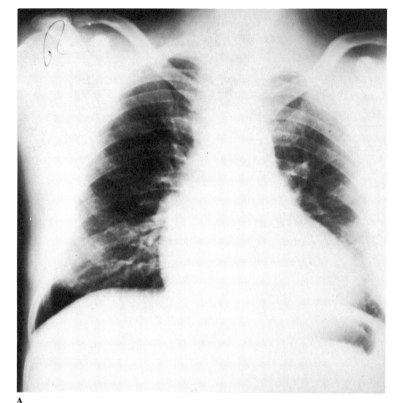

A

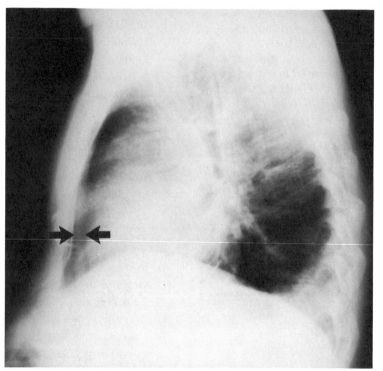

B

**Fig. 5-8.** *Hilar adenopathy is well seen on the right side in this patient with sarcoidosis. The right hilum is large and the margins are not clearly blood vessels (black arrows). The azygos node is enlarged; it is seen above the black arrow on the posteroanterior (PA) view (**A**) projected over the right posterior fifth and sixth ribs. (Marked adenopathy is seen in Fig. 5-33.) A slight pectus excavatum deformity is seen on the lateral projection (**B**). It results in a normal variation on the PA view—fuzziness of the right heart border and adjacent density in the lung (open arrow).*

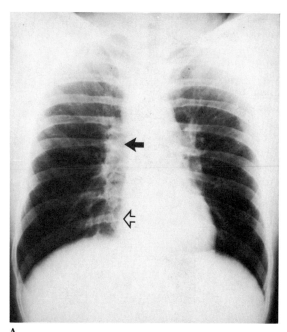

A

B

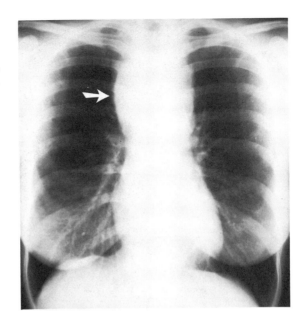

**Fig. 5-9.** *The mediastinal mass (arrow) in this 39-year-old patient was located anteriorly. Most likely causes would be substernal thyroid, thymoma, Hodgkin's disease, or teratoma. This proved to be a thymoma.*

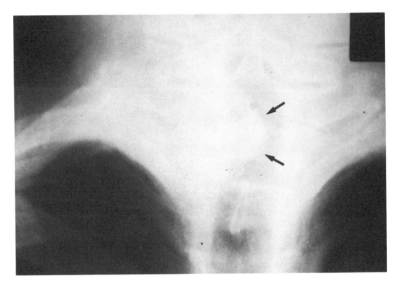

**Fig. 5-10.** *The tracheal lucency always should be inspected. Clinical signs of upper airway obstruction call attention to this area. This patient had carcinoma of the thyroid that invaded and narrowed the trachea (arrows).*

**Fig. 5-11.** *A and B. Common benign findings on chest x-ray. The innominate artery is tortuous (curved solid arrow), there is a large density which had been stable for years, possibly a huge right cardiac fat pad (curved open arrow), and a hiatal hernia with an air-fluid level is seen in the retrocardiac region (black arrows).*

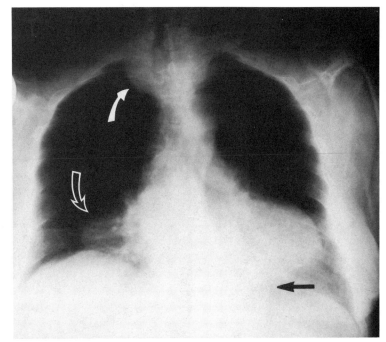

A

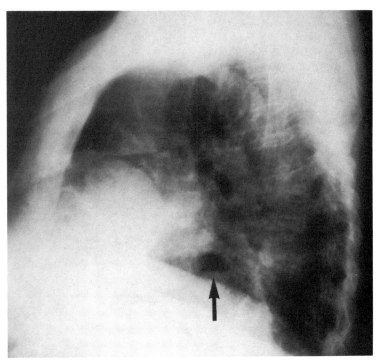

B

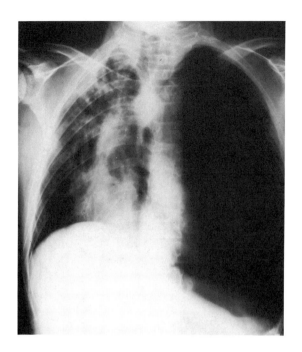

**Fig. 5-12.** *Tension pneumothorax on the left side. The heart and other mediastinal structures are shifted to the right, the left hemidiaphragm is depressed, and the left hemithorax is markedly lucent. Tuberculosis was the cause in this patient.*

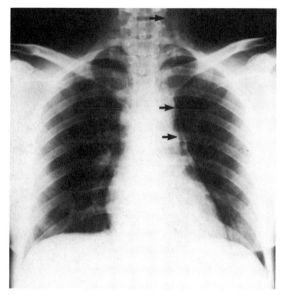

**Fig. 5-13.** *Pneumomediastinum and subcutaneous emphysema. A linear lucency is seen adjacent to the left mediastinum as well as within the soft tissues of the neck (arrows). These are pathognomonic findings.*

**Fig. 5-14.** *The difference in density between the hemithoraces is due to a left radical mastectomy. The normal tissue of the right breast is apparent (long arrows) and is lacking on the left. The postoperative soft tissue defect extends to the left axilla (short arrows).*

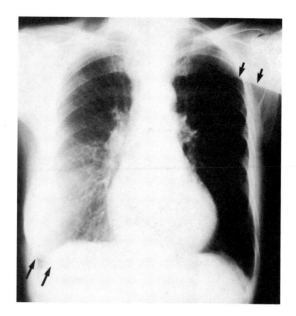

**Fig. 5-15.** *The edges of x-rays should always be checked. Subcutaneous emphysema (arrow) could be overlooked easily in this patient.*

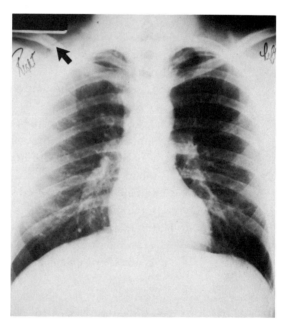

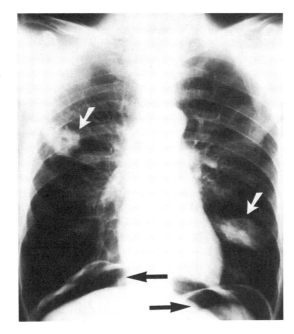

**Fig. 5-16.** *Free intraperitoneal air (black arrows) is well seen on chest x-ray. A ruptured colonic diverticulum was the cause in this patient. Note also the cavitating pseudomonas pneumonia (white arrows).*

## VI. Soft tissues

A. Apparent differential density in the lungs may actually be caused by

1. Asymmetric thoracic soft tissue (e.g., prior mastectomy) (Fig. 5-14)

2. Rotation of the patient (see Fig. 5-2)

B. Subcutaneous emphysema may indicate more serious airway disruption in the neck, in the mediastinum, lungs, or pleura (Fig. 5-15).

C. Cutaneous nevi or raised superficial lesions may simulate intrapulmonary nodules.

D. Infradiaphragmatic soft tissues should be scrutinized for

1. Free air or dilated bowel (Fig. 5-16)

2. Masses or calcifications

THORACIC DISEASES

**I. Pneumonia** (Figs. 5-16, 5-17, 5-18, 5-19, and 5-20). Radiographic characterization of pneumonia has been classified as lobar pneumonia, bronchopneumonia, and mixed. There is overlap on chest x-ray since bacterial, viral, fungal, and even protozoal organisms have varied presentations and appearances.

A. **Patterns**

1. **Consolidation.** Focal increased density.

2. **Lobar.** Increased density conforming to a lobe.

3. **Interstitial.** Normal bronchovascular markings becoming poorly defined because of peribronchial inflammation.

**Fig. 5-17.** *Early* Pneumocystis *pneumonia in a patient with acquired immunodeficiency syndrome. The only findings are poorly defined, fuzzy bronchovascular markings. Early findings may be quite subtle. (Compare the edges of the vessels in the lower lungs with Fig. 5-1.)*

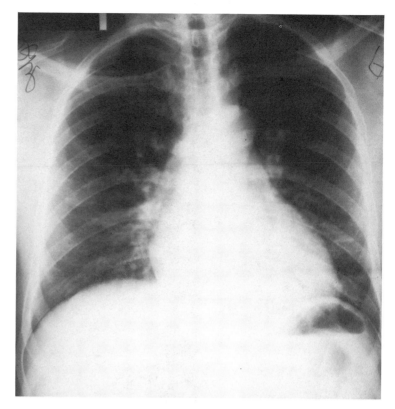

**Fig. 5-18.** *Pneumatoceles in a child. The organism usually is* Staphylococcus. *The pneumatoceles are seen at the left base (arrows). The right upper lobe air-fluid level is a lung abscess.*

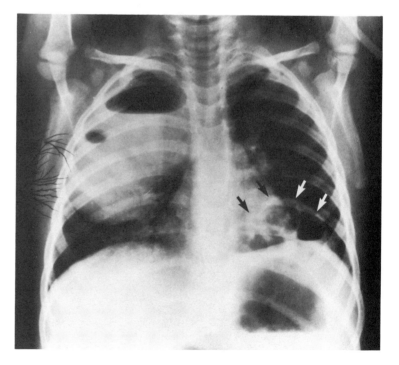

**Fig. 5-19.** *Pneumonia is seen most frequently as poorly marginated areas of focal increased density. The air spaces of the lung filled with fluid and adjacent normal soft tissue structures (such as vessels) are obliterated. Arrows depict the consolidation in the right middle lobe on both posteroanterior (A) and lateral (B) views. There is also a faint "infiltrate" in the lingula just lateral to the cardiac apex.*

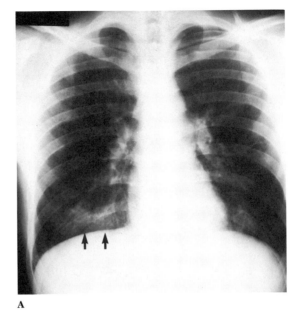

A

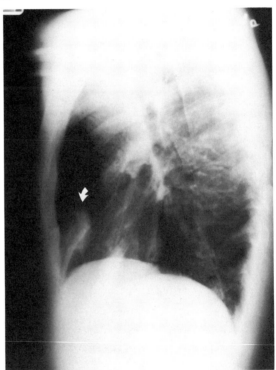

B

**Fig. 5-20.** *Cavitating infarcts due to septic emboli.*

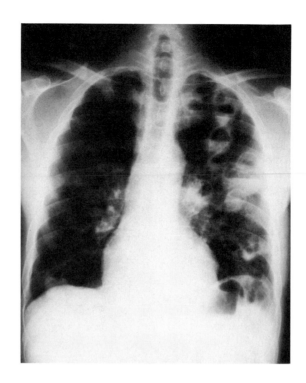

4. **Caveat.** A pectus excavation deformity may simulate right middle lobe pneumonia (Fig. 5-21).

B. **Associated findings**

1. **Pleural effusion and empyema.** More common with *Streptococcus* and gram-negative organisms.

2. **Hilar and/or mediastinal adenopathy.** May be inflammatory adenopathy. May represent an underlying tumor with secondary pneumonia.

3. **Tumor.** A central mass is the clue to an obstructing tumor with peripheral pneumonia; similarly, pneumonia should be followed to radiographic resolution in the appropriate clinical situation to be certain there is not an occult tumor.

4. **Cavitation.** Most common with *Streptococcus,* gram-negative organisms and tuberculosis (tumors occasionally may cavitate as well).

5. **Lung abscess and bronchopleural fistula.** Seen with necrotizing, fulminant, and resistant organisms; abscess is seen most commonly in alcoholic patients with poor dentition.

C. **Types of pneumonia**

1. **Pneumococcus.** The prototype of lobar consolidation
   a. Air bronchograms are common.
   b. May be patchy and multisegmental.

**Fig. 5-21.** *Pitfalls on chest x-ray due to pectus excavatum deformity. The posteroanterior (PA) film alone (**A**) could result in two false-positive diagnoses, cardiomegaly and a right middle lobe pneumonia. The transverse diameter of the heart appears large, and the apex is shifted laterally (small arrow). The right heart border and adjacent vessels are indistinct and there is adjacent density apparently in the lung (large arrow). However, the lateral view (**B**) demonstrates the pronounced pectus deformity (arrow). The heart and lungs are normal on the lateral view.*

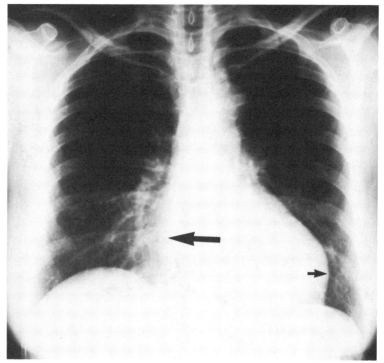

A

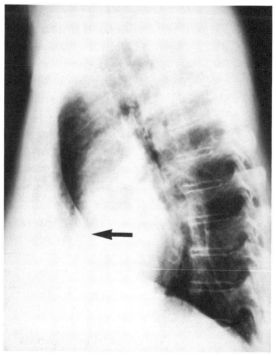

B

## 2. Aspiration

**a.** Typical history is of comatose patient with poor dentition.

**b. Mixed** infections, which commonly include *Bacteroides*.

**c.** Caused by gravity; occurs most frequently in posterior and lower lobes.

## 3. Gram-negative organisms

**a.** Often cause severe infection in an already debilitated patient.

**b.** Common complications include cavitation and empyema.

## 4. Staphylococcal. Often diffuse and rapidly progressive with complicating abscess or pneumatoceles

## 5. Tuberculous. Primary tuberculous pneumonia is uncommon; the primary disease usually is subclinical. The **radiographs** show the following:

**a.** Peripheral, often patchy consolidated infiltrate

**b.** Enlarged hilar nodes

**c.** Geographic or socioeconomic background is clue

## 6. Viral

**a.** Caused by a variety of organisms, most commonly adenovirus. (Others include respiratory syncytial virus, influenza, parainfluenza.)

**b. X-ray findings.** Reticular density, progressing to patchy air-space infiltrate.

**c.** Usually self-limited.

## 7. *Mycoplasma pneumoniae*

**a.** Common form of pneumonia (up to one-third of all pneumonias)

**b. X-ray findings**

(1) Basilar predilection

(2) Reticular pattern early, then patchy infiltrates

(3) Pleural effusion in a minority of cases

## 8. Fungal

**a.** Histoplasmosis and coccidioidomycosis most frequently in the United States

**b. X-ray:** Patchy, fleeting infiltrates often associated with

(1) Hilar adenopathy

(2) Calcified granulomas

## 9. Opportunistic. This group of pneumonias occurs in immunocompromised patients; the infection is caused either by the disease or by immunosuppression owing to therapy.

**a.** Organisms are either common bacteria, viruses, or fungi that overwhelm the host or organisms that rarely

**Fig. 5-22.** *Congestive heart failure (CHF) and pulmonary edema. A. The heart is markedly enlarged. There is edema in the air spaces of the lower lungs; the vessels are obliterated by perivascular edema, and the lungs have excessive density. **B** and **C** were taken following treatment for pulmonary edema. The heart is smaller, although still enlarged. The enlarged left atrium is seen (white arrows). The airspace density has cleared although the vessels in the lungs still look fuzzy, indicating increased interstitial density. (Compare with Fig. 5.1.) With repeated CHF, a chronic interstitial density develops that represents the patient's "baseline." Comparison with old films is critical to decide whether the patient has mild CHF. This patient had a prior mitral valve replacement (black arrow) for mitral stenosis and regurgitation. (The mitral valve is more posterior than the aortic valve.)*

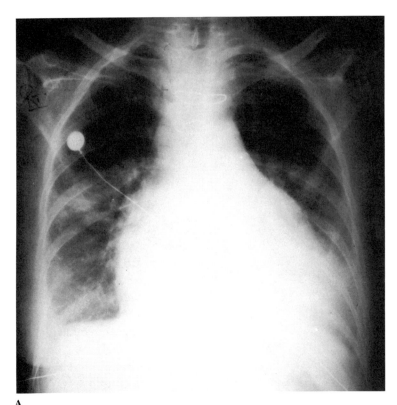

A

cause disease in normal patients (cytomegalovirus, herpesvirus, *Toxoplasma gondii, Nocardia, Aspergillus, Candida, Cryptococcus, Pneumocystis*).

b. These organisms produce a variety of pulmonary, pleural, and hilar findings; there is much overlap and nonspecificity in the findings.

c. Opportunistic pneumonias occur with

　(1) **Neoplastic diseases**—leukemia, lymphoma, carcinoma, sarcoma, myeloma

　(2) **Nonneoplastic diseases**—organ transplantation, diabetes, congenital immune deficiency, acquired immunodeficiency syndrome (AIDS) (pneumocystis and nonspecific pneumonitis most frequent).

II. **Congestive heart failure.** Congestive heart failure (CHF) is a common cause of emergency room visits. There is a spectrum of presentations, from instances that are easy to diagnose clinically to dyspnea of uncertain cause. General considerations:

1. Chest x-ray is valuable in cases of diagnostic difficulty or to monitor response to therapy.

2. Of importance is that the chest x-ray may demonstrate findings before they can be auscultated.

3. A general correlation between pulmonary vascular mani-

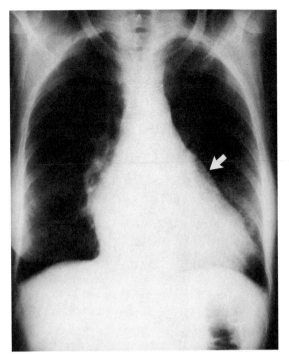

B

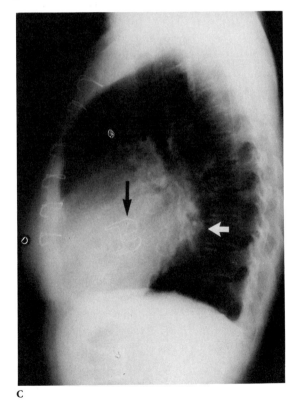

C

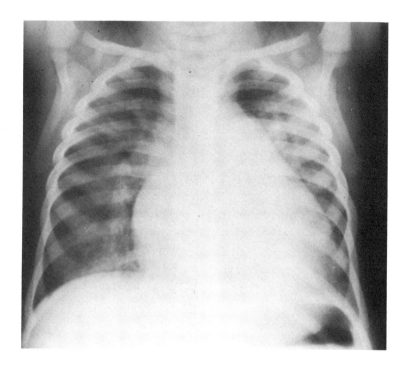

**Fig. 5-23.** *Pulmonary edema in a 3-year-old child. The findings are similar to those in Fig. 5-22A. The etiology in this patient was end-stage renal disease and cardiomyopathy.*

festations of CHF by x-ray and pulmonary wedge pressure may be helpful.

4. Identifying specific cardiac chamber enlargement provides clues to etiologic and underlying pathology.

5. A small heart is an immediate tip-off to the important category of "noncardiogenic pulmonary edema."

6. Old films for comparison are essential.

7. Technical problems from portable x-rays are important in the radiographic evaluation of CHF and are discussed below.

8. *Radiographic findings with CHF* include the following (Figs. 5-22, 5-23, and 5-24):

A. **Vascularity and lungs in CHF**

1. Normally, central and peripheral pulmonary arteries and veins have sharp contours, and gradually taper peripherally. Vessels are larger in the lower lungs than in the upper lungs normally.

2. A sequence of pulmonary vessel changes occurs in CHF: equalization of size of upper and lower vessels, followed by progressive enlargement of the upper lobe vessels (Table 5-2).

3. The hila, normally well defined, become indistinct and enlarge as edema worsens.

B. **The pleura and interstitium in CHF**

1. Pleural effusions are hallmarks of CHF. Right pleural effu-

**Fig. 5-24.** *Interstitial pulmonary edema due to congestive heart failure.* **A** *and* **B.** *There is cardiomegaly and increased interstitial density throughout the lungs. The vessels are ill-defined. Kerley B lines are visible (white arrows) perpendicular to and abutting the pleura. Seen most frequently in the lower lungs, they represent septae distended with fluid. The costophrenic angles are blunted and the major fissure appears thickened (black arrow), both findings indicative of pleural fluid. Following treatment (*C*) the Kerley B lines disappeared and the vessels became better defined.*

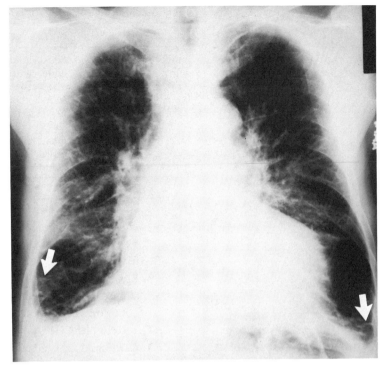

A

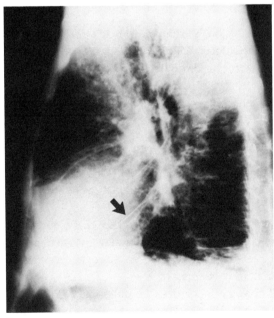

B

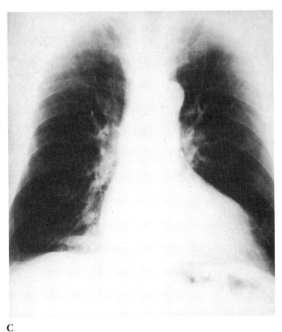

C

**Table 5-2.** *Manifestations of Pulmonary Edema on Chest X-ray*

| Stage of CHF | Chest x-ray finding |
|---|---|
| Pulmonary venous hypertension | Equalization of upper and lower lobe vessel sizes<br>Redistribution—upper lobe vessels larger than lower lobe vessels |
| Interstitial edema | Hilar and bronchovascular markings indistinct<br>Kerley B lines<br>Subpleural fluid "thickens" fissures |
| Alveolar edema | Bilateral perihilar density in "batwing" distribution<br>Pleural effusion(s) (right greater than left) |

sion is usually greater than left, or right effusion is seen alone.

2. Fissure "thickening" from subpleural fluid is an early manifestation of CHF.

3. Kerley lines indicate fluid in interstitial lymphatics and signify elevated wedge pressure; Kerley B lines are most common and reliable.

C. **The heart in CHF**

1. Cardiomegaly is a hallmark of CHF.

2. Left atrial enlargement indicates elevated left-sided cardiac pressures, unless pulmonary edema occurs acutely (uncommon).

3. Pericardial effusion is frequent; when large, it may obscure evaluation of specific cardiac chambers; pericardial effusion is better diagnosed by lateral chest x-ray than by PA or AP views (see Fig. 5-7).

4. Left ventricular aneurysm is another finding that may occur with CHF; a posterior left-sided bulge in the heart, which may calcify is characteristic (Fig. 5-25).

D. **Other clues to CHF**

1. Knowledge that a patient has been in CHF in the past may help clarify a nonspecific finding such as "diffuse interstitial markings."

2. Particularly with mitral disease (especially mitral stenosis), iron and fibrotic deposition may give an abnormal chronic interstitial appearance without the presence of acute pulmonary edema.

3. In CHF, **change** in cardiac or pulmonary findings on x-ray is more important than background radiographic abnormalities.

4. **Caveat.** Chronic interstitial changes due to CHF may mimic acute CHF; old films and heart size are important for differentiation (Figs. 5-22 and 5-26).

E. **Noncardiogenic pulmonary edema** (Fig. 5-27)

**Fig. 5-25.** *Calcified left ventricular aneurysm (arrows) and chronic obstructive pulmonary disease (COPD). The bulging cardiac contour is characteristic of an aneurysm. This patient also has characteristic findings of COPD: flattened diaphragms, increased anteroposterior diameter from hyperexpansion of the lungs, and increased lucency in the lungs. The flattened hemidiaphragms blunt the costophrenic sulci, giving the (false) appearance of pleural effusion.*

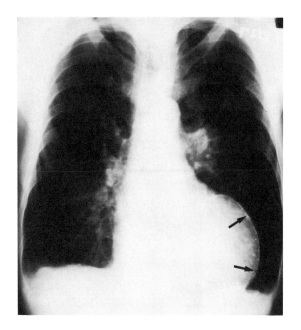

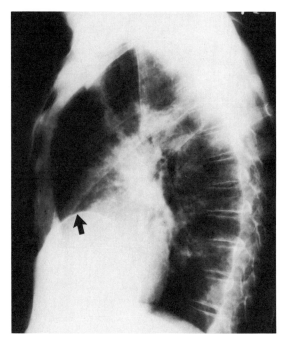

**5. The Chest**

**Fig. 5-26.** *Chronic interstitial lung disease in a patient with pulmonary fibrosis. There is increased interstitial density, indistinct vessels (straight arrows), and thickening of the walls of the larger bronchi seen en face near the hila (curved arrow). Indistinct vascular margins and "peribronchial cuffing" indicate increased interstitial density from any cause and are nonspecific findings.*

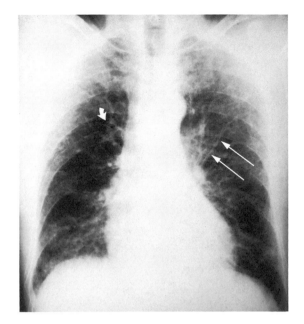

**Fig. 5-27.** *Noncardiogenic pulmonary edema in a patient who had a near drowning in fresh water. The air-space density usually is symmetric. The heart is normal sized.*

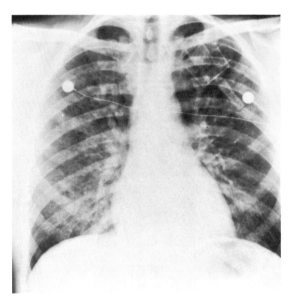

**Table 5-3.** *Causes of Noncardiogenic Pulmonary Edema (normal heart size, pulmonary edema pattern)*

Adult respiratory distress syndrome (ARDS)
Heroin overdose
Inhalation of noxious gases
Near-drowning
High altitude
Fat emboli
Gastric aspiration (Mendelson's syndrome)
Neurogenic pulmonary edema
Pulmonary vein occlusion

1. The clue is a "pulmonary edema pattern" with a normal-sized heart.
2. Causes are summarized in Table 5-3.
3. **Caveat.** The noncardiogenic pattern may occur with acute myocardial infarction when sufficient time has not elapsed to allow left atrial enlargement.

F. **Caveats for interpretation of CHF by portable chest x-ray**

1. Portable films that are taken AP rather than PA result in magnification of anterior chest structures (e.g., the heart).
   a. The heart may appear larger than 50 percent of the thorax in an AP radiograph and still be normal.
   b. The mediastinum and hila also appear spuriously large.
   c. Old films demonstrating sequential cardiac enlargement are more reliable than a single portable chest x-ray.
   d. Comparable technique films should be compared when possible, e.g., PA to PA and AP to AP.
2. Small lung volumes caused by poor inspiration cause apparent vascular and hilar indistinctness, which may falsely simulate interstitial pulmonary edema (see Fig. 5-4).
3. Small lung volumes make the heart appear larger.
4. Supine positioning may cause pleural fluid to layer posteriorly rather than accumulate inferiorly as it usually does on chest x-ray; this may mask a pleural effusion; the clue is hemithorax that appears denser than the contralateral side.

III. **Tumor.** Primary or metastatic lung tumor can prompt an emergency room visit for a variety of reasons (Figs. 5-28, 5-29, 5-30, and 5-31).

A. **Postobstructive pneumonia.** A central mass or large adenopathy may cause atelectasis and subsequent consolidation in the partially collapsed lobe or segment. This requires careful inspection of the perihilar regions for an underlying

**Fig. 5-28.** *Filling of the lung with fluid may occur with bronchial obstruction. This patient had carcinoma obstructing the left main stem bronchus. There is little mediastinal shift. Other causes of an opaque hemithorax frequently involve mediastinal shift. In postpneumonectomy patients, the heart will shift toward the affected side. In massive pleural effusions, the heart may shift away from the effusion.*

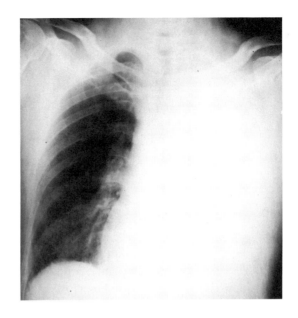

**Fig. 5-29.** *Pulmonary nodule (arrow) representing primary lung carcinoma. The appearance is nonspecific and could be due to benign or malignant causes. Comparison with old films and, if a new finding, fluoroscopic or CT-guided biopsy usually yields a diagnosis.*

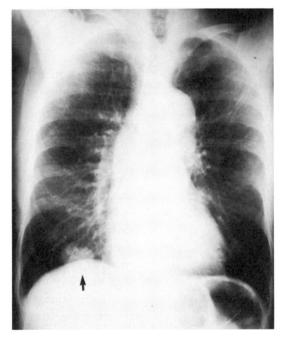

**Fig. 5-30.** *Subtle left apex squamous cell carcinoma. The posteroanterior view (A) and tomogram (B) demonstrate a Pancoast tumor (arrow). The adjacent lung abnormality and bony destruction make this suspicious for tumor rather than benign pleural thickening. The 33-year-old patient had 20 pack-years of smoking, a 6-month history of left shoulder and arm pain, and a 1-week history of left ptosis and miosis (Horner's syndrome).*

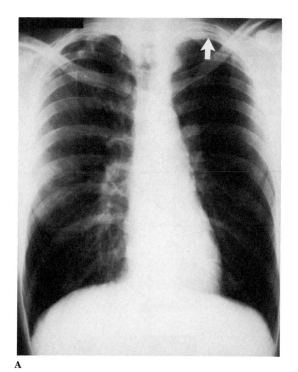

A

B

**Fig. 5-31.** *Metastatic breast carcinoma is the working diagnosis when a large pleural effusion, increased interstitial density (representing lymphangitic spread of tumor), evidence of a mastectomy, and axillary clips are seen.*

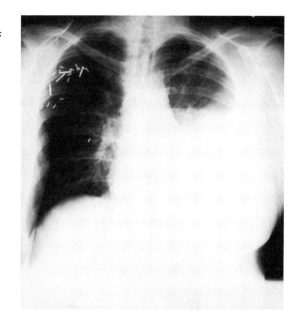

**Fig. 5-32.** *Mesothelioma presenting as a pleural-based mass on the lateral right thorax. The appearance is nonspecific. Further workup includes comparison with old films, CT, and needle biopsy.*

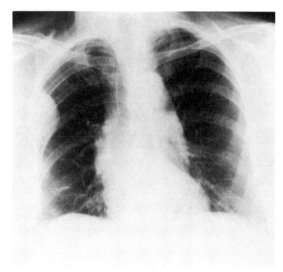

**Fig. 5-33.** *Marked hilar adenopathy (arrows) and interstitial density. This patient has chronic berylliosis; sarcoidosis could have a similar appearance.*

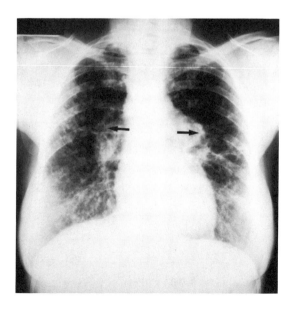

mass and meticulous radiographic follow-up to be certain there is no underlying tumor once the pneumonia has cleared.

**B. Lobar collapse and pleural effusion.** Patients with one or more collapsed lobes or a large pleural effusion may present with dyspnea. Such severe radiographic findings usually occur in patients who have neglected medical care. The underlying tumor mass itself may be obscured by the associated findings.

**C. Pathologic extremity or vertebral rib fracture.** Metastatic bony lesions may fracture and cause pain. Particularly in elderly patients, associated lucency at a new fracture site must be regarded suspiciously as an unsuspected tumor.

**D. Shoulder pain** from a Pancoast (superior sulcus) tumor. Shoulder films obtained for pain may demonstrate an occult tumor in the lung apex. Involvement of the brachial plexus or invasion of ribs may be the cause of the shoulder pain.

**E. Incidental discovery of a nodule or adenopathy.** This may prove lifesaving. Areas to be checked carefully include the apices, perihilar and retrocardiac regions, and lung bases. Calcified nodules usually are benign (old tuberculosis, histoplasmosis).

**IV. Inhalational diseases.** These diseases are caused by chronic or acute exposure to an irritant or agent that causes a hypersensitivity reaction. (Figs. 5-32 and 5-33).

**A.** Agents in occupational exposures that provoke pneumoconioses include silica, asbestos, beryllium, talc, and bauxite.

**B.** Clinically, these patients are chronically dyspneic with exacerbations or secondary infections necessitating emergency room visits.

**C.** Radiographic manifestations vary, depending on the agent

  **1.** Most frequently an interstitial pattern, which may include pulmonary nodules and lines.

  **2.** Bilateral adenopathy occurs with silica and beryllium; these may calcify.

  **3.** Pleural plaques are characteristic of asbestos and talc exposure; these may calcify.

**D.** Asbestosis is associated with mesothelioma and bronchogenic carcinoma, especially in a patient with a history of smoking.

**E.** Barium, tin, coal dust, and iron oxide are relatively benign when inhaled.

**F.** Inhalational diseases may cause emphysematous hyperexpansion of the lungs or end-stage, fibrotic restrictive lungs.

**V. Miscellaneous pulmonary disorders**

**A.** Allergic hypersensitivity diseases (Fig. 5-34). These diseases

**Fig. 5-34.** *Allergic pneumonitis. There is patchy increased density peripherally in the left lung. History and clinical course distinguish allergic pneumonitis from other pneumonias. The allergic pneumonitis was due to a dirty humidifier; it cleared after the humidifier was cleaned.*

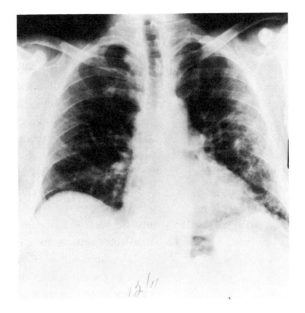

**Fig. 5-35.** *Acute radiation pneumonitis. This 43-year-old female developed cough and dyspnea following treatment with 6400 rads for carcinoma involving the trachea and right lung. The air-space density (arrow) that results from acute radiation treatment corresponds to the radiation port. Note the branching "air bronchograms" (patent bronchi) within the medial portion of this consolidation. Normal lucencies between vessels as seen behind the left side of the heart may mistakenly be called air bronchograms. Air bronchograms are abnormal and are branching air tubes as opposed to vessels, which are branching densities.*

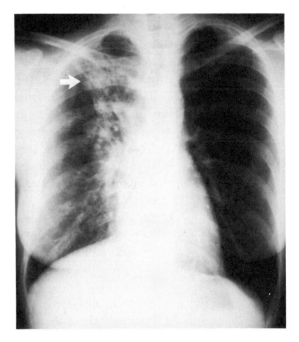

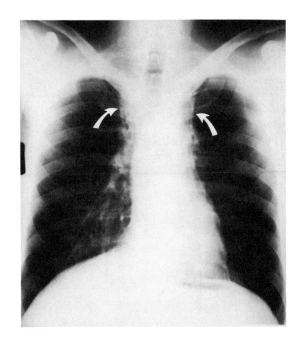

**Fig. 5-36.** *Chronic fibrosis (arrows) from radiation treatment. The radiation port and signs of volume loss are visible post radiation therapy for Hodgkin's disease 12 years previously. Upward retraction of the hila bilaterally represents loss of lung volume in the upper lobes.*

are typically acute, and characterized by dyspnea. There may be fever, chills, and toxicity.

1. Allergens and diseases include grain or hay in farmer's lung disease, dust from cotton, sugar cane extract, maple-bark disease, and pituitary snuff disease.
2. The mechanism is inhalation of the allergen.
3. Dyspnea, prostration, and fever occur acutely, although exposure may have occurred for several months.
4. X-ray findings include localized or diffuse poorly defined infiltrates.

B. Radiation pneumonitis (Figs. 5-35 and 5-36)
1. This occurs in cancer patients who have received 4500 to 6000 rads.
2. The interval between radiation therapy and onset of pneumonitis typically is 4 to 6 weeks.
3. Clinically, patients present with dyspnea, cough, and fever.
4. X-ray acutely reveals a poorly defined area of density corresponding to the radiation port.
5. Chronic x-ray findings include fibrotic stranding with retraction and pleural thickening.

C. Adverse effects of medications (Fig. 5-37)
1. An acute syndrome may occur with nitrofurantoin or penicillin.
2. Clinically, there is fever, cough, dyspnea, and chills; eosinophilia may occur.
3. A chronic syndrome with interstitial fibrosis on chest x-ray occurs with busulfan and methotrexate.

**Fig. 5-37.** *Eosinophilic pneumonia due to nitrofurantoin. There is diffuse interstitial density similar to interstitial pulmonary edema or pulmonary fibrosis. In acute toxicity the lungs rapidly return to normal after cessation of the drug. Occasionally a chronic form develops.*

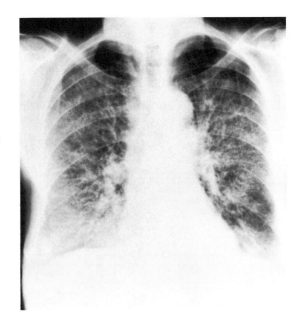

**Fig. 5-38.** *Salt-water drowning: bilateral diffuse air-space disease. The appearance is not distinguishable from fresh-water drowning, other causes of pulmonary edema, or severe pneumonia.*

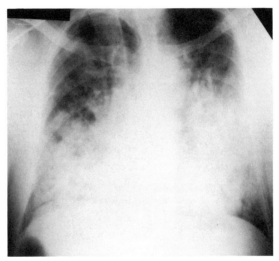

**Fig. 5-39.** *Findings of pericardial effusion with cardiac tamponade, and air-space density consistent with pulmonary edema. This patient had systemic lupus erythematosus.*

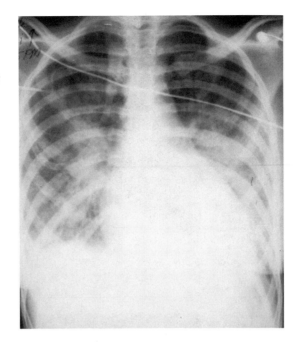

**Fig. 5-40.** *Wegener's granulomatosis in this 28-year-old patient presented as a solitary somewhat nodular density (arrow). Usually there are multiple bilateral widely distributed nodules. Cavitation of nodules occurs in one-third to one-half of cases.*

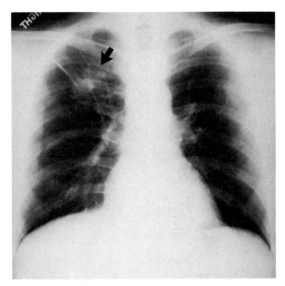

**Fig. 5-41.** *Chronic eosinophilic pneumonia is characterized by peripheral nonsegmental homogeneous consolidation. The appearance is identical to Loeffler's syndrome, although the consolidations tend to persist for days or weeks in contrast to the more migratory appearance in Loeffler's.*

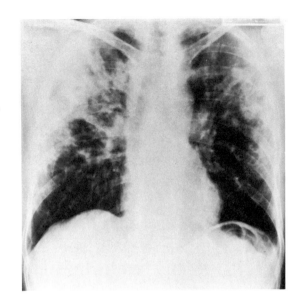

**Fig. 5-42.** *Adult respiratory distress syndrome (ARDS) has a variable appearance that may be radiographically similar to pulmonary edema. In this patient the heart size is normal. ARDS describes a clinical rather than radiographic picture of acute severe respiratory distress in patients with or without underlying lung disease.*

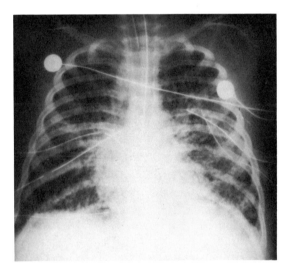

**D. Near-drowning.** Pulmonary edema with a normal-sized heart is the radiographic finding with salt water near-drowning (Fig. 5-38).

**E. Immune connective tissue diseases** (Figs. 5-39 and 5-40). The various disorders in this broad category have markedly different appearances. The major characteristics follow:

    **1. Systemic lupus erythematosus** (SLE). Pleural and pericardial effusions are most common; parenchymal changes are multiple and patchy.

    **2. Wegener's granulomatosis.** Characterized by thick-walled cavitating nodules; there is associated thickening of the paranasal sinuses.

    **3. Rheumatoid arthritis.** The most frequent findings are diffuse fibrosis, nodules (which often cavitate), and pleural effusions.

    **4. Scleroderma.** Characteristic finding is bibasilar fibrosis.

**F. PIE syndrome.** This group of diseases is characterized by pulmonary infiltrates with eosinophilia. Patients may present in the emergency setting with the following (Fig. 5-41):

    **1. Loeffler's syndrome.** Self-limited fleeting infiltrates with a mild respiratory illness.

    **2. Chronic eosinophilic pneumonia.** A more severe entity with a chronic nature unless recognized.

        **a.** The infiltrates are changeable and have a propensity for upper outer portions of the lungs (axillary segments).

        **b.** Response to steroids is often dramatic.

    **3.** A variant is associated with asthma.

**G. Adult respiratory distress syndrome** (Fig. 5-42)

    **1.** Nonspecific entity caused by a variety of insults, including trauma, infection, and environmental agents.

    **2.** Patient usually is critically ill and has been hospitalized.

    **3.** Pulmonary edema pattern appears on chest x-ray, often with a small heart.

SELECTED READINGS

Benacerraf BR, McLoud TC, Rhea JT, et al. Assessment of the contribution of chest radiography in outpatients with acute chest complaints: A prospective study. Radiology 138:293, 1981.

Findley LJ, Sahn SA. Value of chest roentgenograms in acute asthma in adults. Chest 80:535, 1981.

Greene R. Screening chest radiography: Its role in modern medicine. Australas Radiol 26:10, 1982.

Hubbell FA, Greenfield S, Tyler JL, et al. Impact of routine admission chest x-rays on patient care. Radiology 156:853, 1985.

Kattan KR. Some telltales and pitfalls in chest radiology. Radiol Clin North Am 22:467, 1984.

Klein DL. Visibility of the inferior heart border in pneumoperitoneum. AJR 137:622, 1981.

Rhea JT, vanSonnenberg E, McLoud T. Basilar pneumothorax in the supine adult. Radiology 133:593, 1979.

Smith R, Ellis K, Alderson PO. Role of chest radiography in predicting the extent of airway disease in patients with suspected pulmonary embolism. Radiology 159:391, 1986.

Young JWR, Andersen BL, Keinig JW. Oblique chest film: Value in routine and selective use. AJR 142:69, 1984.

# 6  The Abdomen

*Eric vanSonnenberg and James T. Rhea*

This chapter is divided into two sections. The first section describes an orderly method for reviewing plain abdominal films in the emergency room setting. It describes normal structures, variations, and general categories of abnormalities, serving as a checklist to ensure that all aspects of the radiograph are perused. The second section includes specific diseases and their radiographic findings.

SYSTEMATIC VIEWING METHOD

I. **Gas/air.** These terms are used interchangeably; most accurately, however, it is gas in the gastrointestinal tract, composed primarily of carbon dioxide. **Three categories of abnormal gas** should be checked for: (1) free or retroperitoneal air, (2) bowel gas pattern, and (3) pathologic gas.

A. **Free air (pneumoperitoneum)** usually signifies **perforation** of a hollow viscus.

1. *Most frequent causes:* **perforated duodenal ulcer, perforated stomach** (ulcer or tumor), **perforation of the cecum or small bowel.**

2. **Absence of free air does not exclude perforation.**

3. Perforation of the appendix or colonic diverticula usually is not associated with free air.

4. **Benign (clinically insignificant) free air** may occur under the following circumstances:

 a. Postoperatively (up to 7 days)

 b. Postparacentesis

 c. After dialysis or any intraperitoneal catheter insertion

 d. After vaginal douching

 e. Associated with "benign" pneumatosis cystoides intestinalis

 f. Idiopathically

5. **Radiographic findings of pneumoperitoneum**

 a. Best seen on **upright abdominal or chest x-rays** as a **closely applied lucency immediately below the hemidiaphragm** (Fig. 6-1).

 b. In patients who cannot be placed in an upright position, a **lateral decubitus view** (preferably left side down) or **cross-table lateral** view (supine patient) will demonstrate free air. Keeping the patient in the

183

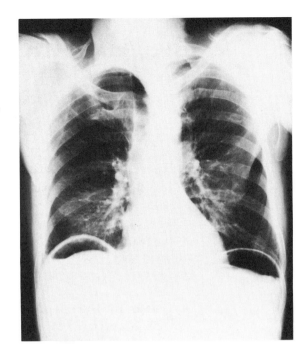

**Fig. 6-1.** *Pneumoperitoneum. Upright abdominal or chest film demonstrates pathognomonic lucencies conforming to the undersurfaces of the hemidiaphragms. Gastric or colonic gas must be differentiated; they have internal wall markings.*

desired position for **10 minutes** will increase accumulation of air and improve visualization (Fig. 6-2).

**c.** Free air under the left hemidiaphragm must be differentiated from the stomach and splenic flexure of the colon.

**d.** Visualization of free air on **supine films** (Fig. 6-3)

    **(1)** Lucency on **both sides of bowel wall**

    **(2)** Lucency outlining the **falciform ligament** in the right upper quadrant

    **(3)** Central **large round lucency** in the midabdomen (especially in children)

    **(4)** Sharp demarcation of intraperitoneal organs (liver, gallbladder, spleen)

**B. Retroperitoneal gas** (Fig. 6-4) is **not** free air and is not intraperitoneal.

  **1.** Causes

    **a.** Most frequently, perforation of the retroperitoneal duodenum or ascending and descending colon.

    **b.** Renal or perirenal abscesses.

    **c.** Perforation of the rectum may dissect upward into the retroperitoneum.

    **d.** Conversely, mediastinal gas may dissect inferiorly into the retroperitoneum.

  **2.** Radiographic findings

    **a.** Accentuation of renal and psoas margins caused by abnormal lucency.

**Fig. 6-2.** *Pneumoperitoneum. Cross-table lateral or decubitus views are alternatives to upright films.* **A.** *Gas outside the bowel wall accentuates visualization of the wall (white arrows). There is also gas dissecting outside the peritoneal cavity (black arrow).* **B.** *Free intraperitoneal air outlines the falciform ligament (arrow). In addition, the gallbladder is seen because of the free air adjacent to it.*

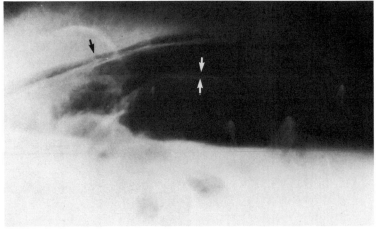

A

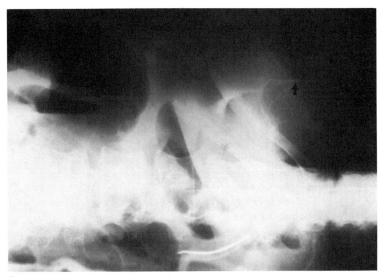

B

**Fig. 6-3.** *Pneumoperitoneum. Free air highlights visualization of the walls of the hepatic flexure and transverse colon (black arrows). The loops of dilated small bowel on the left are closely applied to each other. The density between the air in these loops is the normal thickness of two adjacent bowel walls (white arrows).*

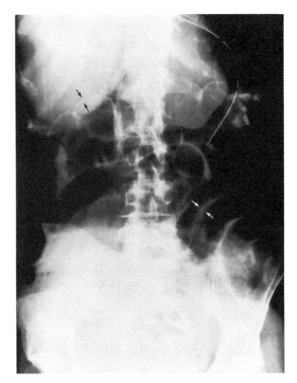

**Fig. 6-4.** *Retroperitoneal gas. The characteristic appearance is streaky and mottled as in the right mid and upper abdomen. Accentuation of the liver edge because of adjacent air is also present.*

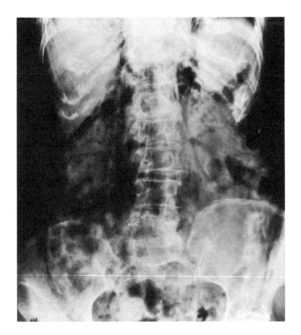

**b.** Mottled, streaky gas often courses up the mediastinum or into soft tissues.

**c.** Position change does not alter appearance of retroperitoneal gas, as with free intraperitoneal gas.

## C. Bowel gas

**1.** Guidelines for dispersal and width of bowel

    **a.** Every intestinal loop cannot be identified and differentiated (small versus large bowel).

    **b.** Air-fluid levels normally occur in the stomach, duodenal bulb, and large intestine (if recent enema administration).

    **c.** Normal amount of gas:

        **(1)** Stomach and large intestine: mild-to-moderate amount fairly evenly dispersed.

        **(2)** Small bowel: minimal to none.

    **d.** Normal luminal diameter

        **(1)** Small bowel—less than 2.5 to 3.0 cm (so-called rule of thumb; if the small intestine is wider than the length of the observer's distal phalanx of the thumb [normally 2.5–3.0 cm], the organ is dilated).

        **(2)** Large bowel—4 cm; the cecum may be up to 6 cm.

    **e.** Bowel wall thickness

        **(1)** Seen when loops are adjacent.

        **(2)** Normal bowel wall is pencil-thin (2–3 mm).

        **(3) Thickened bowel wall** signifies *edema, blood, or tumor* in the wall, fluid between the loops, or loops more than half filled with fluid.

**2. Abnormal bowel gas patterns** (Table 6-1)

    **a. Aerophagia** (Fig. 6-5), or "air-swallowing"

        **(1)** Excess gas in a diffuse minimally dilated pattern throughout the stomach and small and large intestines

        **(2) Causes.** pain, anxiety, crying in infants

    **b. Ileus** (Fig. 6-5)

        **(1)** *Adynamic ileus* and *paralytic ileus* are synonymous.

        **(2) Causes. Inflammatory** (appendicitis, cholecystitis, diverticulitis, pancreatitis, diffuse peritonitis); **vascular** (ischemic); and **metabolic** (hypokalemia, hypocalcemia, hypomagnesemia).

        **(3)** Diffuse (global dilatation of stomach, and small and large intestines) or focal (localized dilatation).

        **(4)** Characteristic (but not exclusive) types of ileus with acute pancreatitis

Table 6-1. *Analysis of Bowel Gas Patterns: Obstruction Versus Paralytic Ileus*

| Diagnosis | Distribution of gas | Dilatation of bowel | Appearance of air-fluid levels (evidence of peristalsis) |
|---|---|---|---|
| **Diagnosis is certain** | | | |
| Normal | No small bowel gas | No dilatation | Present |
| Obstruction (e.g., adhesions, tumor) | Gas seen in continuity proximal to a point with no gas distally | Dilated proximal to a point with proportionate dilatation | Present (air-fluid levels at different heights in same loop of bowel; multiple air-fluid levels) |
| Obstruction (e.g., closed-loop obstruction) | Variable | A loop or adjacent loops are diluted way out of proportion to all other gas | Present, absent, or uncertain |
| **Diagnosis is uncertain** | | | |
| Probably obstruction | Gas throughout bowel | Dilated proximal to a point, less gas in nondilated bowel distally | Present (early obstruction, partial obstruction), absent (partial obstruction, ileus), or uncertain |
| Probably colonic obstruction | Variable | Variable | Air-fluid levels in colon distal to cecum in absence of diarrhea or enemas |
| Probably ileus | Variable (single loop-focal ileus; gas throughout bowel—generalized ileus) | **Moderate** dilatation usually | Absent (air-fluid levels at same height in same loop; fewer air-fluid levels) |
| Probably aerophagia | Small and large bowel gas present | Abundant gas but no significant dilatation | Present |
| Abnormal nonspecific bowel gas pattern | Moderate amounts of small bowel gas | Little or no dilatation | Present, absent, or uncertain |

Notes: Loops dilated with fluid imply obstruction. (May be difficult to recognize on plain films.) Rectal obstruction is usually a probable, not a certain plain film diagnosis, since clearing of gas distally cannot be seen and peristalsis may be absent in any obstruction after a period of time. Analysis of bowel gas patterns, except for the preceding "certain" diagnoses, is judgmental. Experience helps with such qualitative factors as "multiple" versus "few" air-fluid levels, the "degree" of dilatation, and whether dilatation of different parts of the bowel is "proportionate."

**Fig. 6-5. A.** *Abundant gas is seen in nondilated small bowel. The patient was anxious, and the appearance represented aerophagia. An early ileus or distal small bowel obstruction could appear this way. Follow-up films will help to decide.* **B.** *Diffuse ileus. Both large and small bowel are dilated to a moderate degree. Dilatation may not be uniform; as in this patient, the transverse colon is relatively more dilated than the cecum. Ileus cannot be differentiated from obstruction with a single image.*

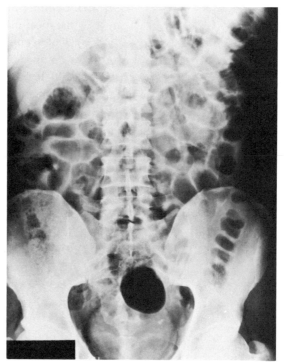

A

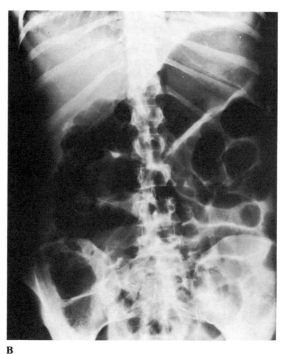

B

(a) "Sentinel loop"—duodenal or proximal jejunal focal dilatation

(b) "Colon cutoff"—focal transverse colon dilatation up to distal splenic flexure

(5) Air-fluid levels may be seen with ileus but are more prominent with obstruction.

(6) **Caveat.** Follow-up films are frequently pivotal in differentiation of ileus from obstruction.

c. **Mechanical small bowel obstruction** (Fig. 6-6)

(1) **Disproportionate** small bowel dilatation compared to large bowel

(2) **Partial versus complete small bowel obstruction**—some versus no gas in large intestine

(3) **Radiographic findings**

(a) The classic **triad**

(i.) Proximal bowel dilation

(ii.) Absence of gas distal to obstruction

(iii.) Evidence of peristaltic activity (multiple air-fluid levels at different heights)

(b) Closed loop obstruction: single loop of bowel distended out of proportion to the remainder of the bowel (*e.g.,* volvulus).

(c) Distended small bowel loops filled with fluid may be seen.

(d) **High small bowel obstruction** (duodenal or jejunal) has minimal to no gas in the distal jejunum, ileum, and large intestine (Fig. 6-7).

(e) Gas below the inguinal ligament signifies a hernia.

(f) **Causes.** Adhesions, internal or external hernias, tumors, gallstones, inflammation (e.g., appendicitis), intramural hemorrhage.

(4) Studies to differentiate obstruction from ileus

(a) Follow-up films

(b) Barium or water-soluble studies

(5) Enemas, sigmoidoscopy, or rectal examination may retrogradely introduce colonic gas, giving the appearance of partial small bowel obstruction (SBO) when there is complete SBO.

d. **Large bowel obstruction** (Fig. 6-8)

(1) Radiographic findings

(a) Dilated large intestine without much small bowel gas (competent ileocecal valve) or with copious small intestinal gas (incompetent ileocecal valve).

(b) The cecum frequently is the most dilated portion of the large intestine (Laplace's law).

**Fig. 6-6.** *Mechanical small bowel obstruction. Note that the small bowel is disproportionately dilated relative to the colon (A), implying a fairly early obstruction or partial obstruction. The upright film shows evidence of peristaltic activity because air-fluid levels are at different heights in the same loop of bowel and there are multiple air-fluid levels throughout the abdomen (B).*

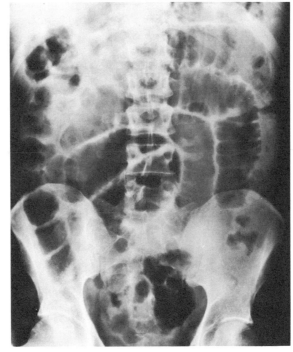

A

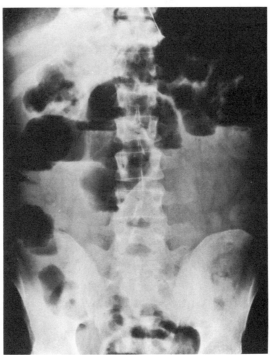

B

**Fig. 6-7.** *Proximal small bowel obstruction. The jejunum is dilated and there is almost no gas distally ( A ). The stomach has been decompressed by a nasogastric tube. The air-fluid levels on the upright film do not imply peristaltic activity since they are not at different heights within the same loop ( B ). In late obstruction, the bowel may quit peristaltic activity. The appearance could represent a focal ileus, although the marked dilatation and absence of distal gas favor obstruction.*

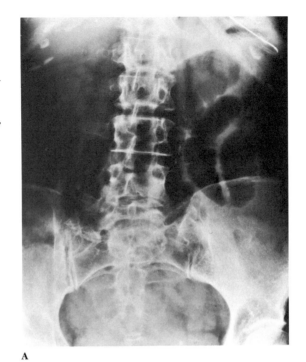

A

B

**Fig. 6-8.** *Large bowel obstruction. There is dilated bowel proximal to the point of obstruction (arrow), no gas distal to the obstruction, and there is evidence of peristaltic activity. The ileocecal valve is incompetent in this patient, resulting in passive dilatation of the small bowel.*

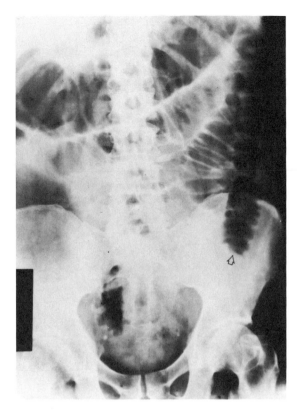

    **(c)** No gas distal to the obstruction.

  **(2)** The **cecum** is the **area most prone to rupture** (greater than *12 cm* diameter is the **danger point**).

  **(3)** **Prone lateral rectum** radiograph demonstrates whether gas passes antegradely into the rectosigmoid. This helps **differentiate large bowel obstruction from ileus.**

  **(4)** Upper gastrointestinal (GI) series with barium is contraindicated with large bowel obstruction—barium may impact in the colon because of the desiccating effect of the large intestine. (Barium may be used safely to demonstrate the point of obstruction with small bowel obstruction.)

**e. Pseudoobstruction of the large intestine** (Ogilvie's syndrome)

  **(1)** Seen in elderly patients who use cathartics and in those taking drugs producing hypotonia (especially antiparkinsonian medications) or with electrolyte abnormalities

  **(2)** May be associated with abdominal pain

  **(3)** Radiographic findings

    **(a)** Dilated, boggy large intestine

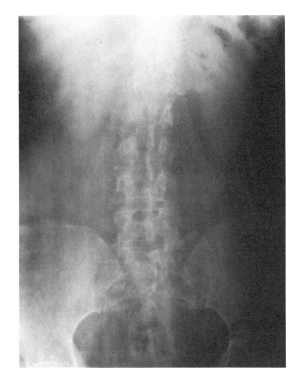

**Fig. 6-9.** *"Gasless abdomen." There is almost complete lack of intestinal gas in this patient who had pancreatitis. The clinical setting helps differentiate normal variation, obstruction with fluid-filled loops, bowel infarction with fluid-filled loops, and pancreatitis.*

        **(b) No** mechanical obstruction

    **f. "Gasless abdomen"** ( Fig. 6-9 )

        **(1)** Minimal to no abdominal gas

        **(2)** Causes

            **(a)** Late small bowel obstruction ( loops are fluid-filled ).

            **(b)** Pancreatitis or mesenteric embolus and bowel infarction.

            **(c)** Occasionally it is an insignificant normal variant.

**D. Pathological gas. Subserosal**

    **1.** Linear or bubbly **intramural gas** ( within the intestinal wall ) ( Fig. 6-10 )

    **2.** Causes

        **a. Benign** pneumatosis cystoides intestinalis ( idiopathic )

        **b. Significant** pneumatosis cystoides intestinalis

            **(1)** Indicates microperforation of mucosa

            **(2)** Seen with **mesenteric vascular infarction, necrotizing entercolitis** in infants, **toxic megacolon** of inflammatory colitis, and **strangulated closed loop obstruction**

    **3. Portal venous gas** ( Fig. 6-11 )

        **a.** An ominous sign, often heralding death

        **b.** Branching intrahepatic gas, located **peripherally** in smaller vessels

**Fig. 6-10.** *Intramural gas (pneumatosis cystoides intestinalis). Gas in the bowel wall is recognized as linear lucent streaks separated from intraluminal gas by a thin density representing the inner portion of the bowel wall (arrows). The gas in the wall has similar lucency to intraluminal gas. Fat adjacent to the bowel is not as lucent as gas; it is separated from intraluminal gas by the full thickness of the bowel wall.*

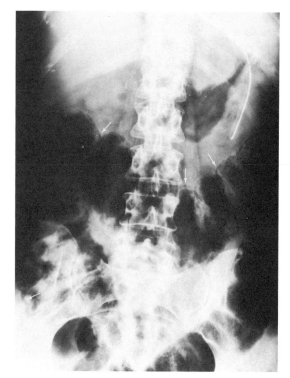

**Fig. 6-11.** *Portal venous gas. Characteristically, the gas is seen best in peripheral veins. This peripheral distribution helps differentiate portal vein gas from bile duct gas (see Fig. 6-12). This finding is seen most frequently with ischemic and infarcted bowel.*

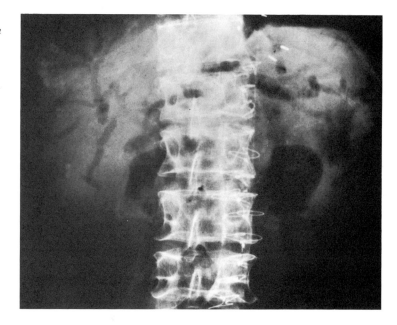

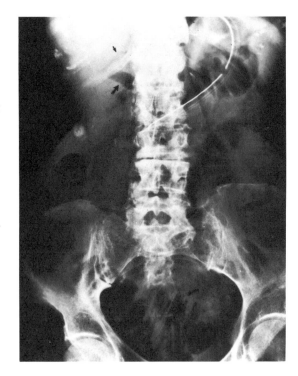

**Fig. 6-12.** *Biliary gas. Gas in bile ducts is more centrally located than portal venous gas. Gas is seen in the main (large straight arrow) and the left hepatic ducts (small straight arrow) in this patient. This patient also has dilated loops of small bowel (curved arrow) with little gas in the colon, findings suggesting small bowel obstruction. In the appropriate clinical setting the combination of gas in bile ducts and small bowel obstruction suggests the possibility of "gallstone ileus." The gallstone may be seen as well, but has passed per rectum in this patient.*

    **c.** Causes

        **(1)** Bowel infarct in adults

        **(2)** Necrotizing enterocolitis in infants

**4. Biliary gas** ( Fig. 6-12)

    **a.** Usually in **central,** large bile ducts (common and left hepatic ducts)

    **b.** Etiology

        **(1)** Postoperative biliary-enteric bypass

        **(2)** Gallstone fistula into stomach, duodenum, or right colon

        **(3)** Emphysematous cholecystitis and cholangitis from gas-producing organism

**5. Abscess** ( Fig. 6-13 )

    **a. Radiographically**

        **(1)** Bubbly and mottled

        **(2)** Well-defined extraintestinal gas collection

        **(3)** Usually ill-defined gas and a circumscribed mass is not apparent

    **b. Caveat.** The cecum, ascending colon, and rectum may normally have a mottled appearance.

**6. Gas-forming infections within viscera**

    **a. Emphysematous cholecystitis, pyelonephritis, and cystitis**

        **(1)** Usually in diabetics caused by gram-negative organisms.

**Fig. 6-13.** *Pathological gas. This patient has gas in a distended gallbladder (large arrows), and in an adjacent abscess (small arrows). A bubbly and mottled appearance is characteristic, but must be differentiated from colonic gas.*

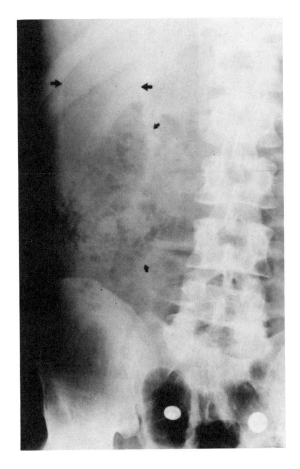

(2) Gas can be intramural, in the lumen, or adjacent to the viscera (Fig. 6-14).

b. **Intrahepatic abscess.** Mottled gas, possible fluid level in the liver (Fig. 6-15)

c. **Subphrenic, subhepatic, lesser sac, pelvic abscesses**

(1) **Mottled extraluminal gas** or air-fluid level in a mass

(2) Adjacent bowel displacement and, commonly, adjacent ileus

II. **Organ outlines.** The liver, spleen, kidney, and bladder should be visualized routinely and checked for size and configuration. Each is seen because of surrounding fat or adjacent gas that has a different density from the organ.

A. **Liver.** Signs of enlargement (Fig. 6-16)

1. Margin below iliac crest on supine film with a medial convex bulging border.

2. Epigastric extension of liver signifies left lobe enlargement or mass.

3. Displacement of hepatic flexure inferiorly; displacement of stomach to the left and posteriorly due to left lobe enlargement.

**Fig. 6-14.** *Emphysematous cho-lecystitis. The large rounded collection of gas in the right upper quadrant proved to be in the gallbladder in this diabetic patient.*

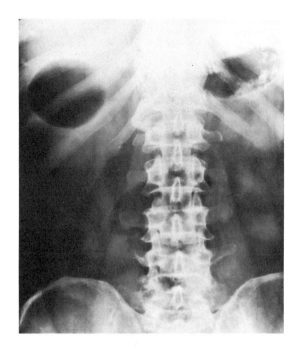

**Fig. 6-15.** *Gas in abscesses. Mottled lucencies are seen in the liver and immediately below the right diaphragm in this patient with intrahepatic and subphrenic abscesses (arrows).*

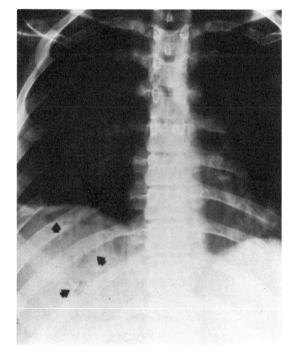

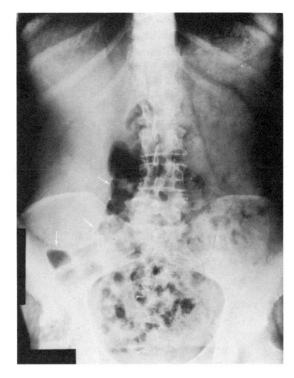

**Fig. 6-16.** *Hepatomegaly is characterized by the presence of a convex portion of the liver below the iliac crest on a supine film (arrows). Note the inferior and medial displacement of the ascending colon and hepatic flexure.*

**4.** Elevated right hemidiaphragm.

**5. Caveat.** Riedel's lobe is a thin, inferior extension of the right lobe. It is a normal variant and can mimic an enlarged liver (Fig. 6-17).

**B. Splenic** enlargement

    **1.** Inferior margin below the twelfth rib on supine film.

    **2.** Stomach displaced medially, splenic flexure inferiorly.

    **3.** Elevation of the left hemidiaphragm.

    **4. Caveat.** Subcapsular fluid or infiltrative diseases in the spleen (or liver) cannot be distinguished from overall organ enlargement on plain films.

**C. Kidneys** (plain film and intravenous urogram [IVU] findings) (Fig. 6-17)

    **1. Size** (9.5–14 cm)

        **a.** Somewhat larger in males than females.

        **b.** Generally symmetric or within 2 cm of each other.

        **c.** Large kidneys occur normally with duplicated systems.

    **2. Axis**

        **a.** Upper poles tilt medially, parallel to the psoas margins.

        **b.** Vertical or lateral position of the upper pole suggests renal displacement by an intrinsic renal mass or extrinsic mass (adrenal, lymph node, fluid collection).

        **c.** Horseshoe or fused kidneys have abnormal axes (vertical axis or lateral tilt of upper poles).

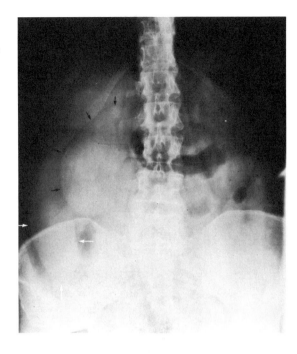

**Fig. 6-17.** *The thin Riedel's lobe is a normal hepatic variation; it extends inferior to the iliac crest (white arrows). It is not as wide or bulging in appearance as is hepatomegaly. (Compare with Fig. 6-16.) The kidneys are well seen because of adjacent fat (black arrows).*

3. **Contour**
   a. Diffuse or focal irregularity indicates scarring from chronic pyelonephritis or renal infarct.
   b. Focal masses are usually renal cysts or hypernephromas (the former are more lucent).
4. **Nonvisualization**
   a. May be because of **congenital** or **surgical absence.**
   b. **Congenital absence** involves contralateral **compensatory enlargement** of the normal solitary kidney.
5. **IV contrast (IVU)**
   a. Visualization of the nephrogram should occur within 1 to 2 minutes.
   b. Collecting systems are seen within 3 minutes.
   c. Nonvisualization after contrast indicates nonfunction, ectopic kidneys, or acute obstruction.

D. **Bladder**
   1. **The most frequent cause of a pelvic mass is an enlarged bladder.**
   2. To distinguish the bladder from a pelvic mass radiographically, the patient must void or the bladder outline must be seen as distinct from the mass (Fig. 6-18). (If uncertainty persists, ultrasound is the procedure of choice.)

E. **Gallbladder**
   1. Not seen routinely.
   2. Enlargement presents as right upper quadrant or right midabdominal mass.

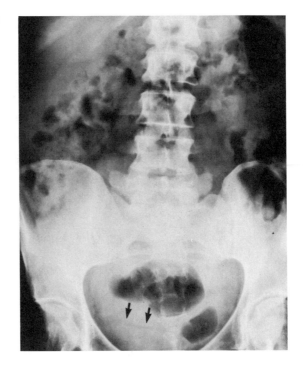

**Fig. 6-18.** *The bladder. The dome of the bladder usually is distinguished from the uterus or a pelvic mass (as in this patient) because of perivesicular fat (arrows). To further define the bladder, a repeat film following voiding or a sonogram may be obtained.*

3. Causes of enlargement (Fig. 6-19)
   a. Hydrops with cystic duct obstruction
   b. Courvoisier gallbladder (biliary obstruction caused by tumor)
   c. Acalculous cholecystitis
   d. Abscess

III. **Masses**
   A. **Pseudomasses**
      1. Fluid-filled viscera or bowel including the bladder, gastric fundus, duodenal bulb, small bowel loops, cecum, and portions of the sigmoid colon
      2. May be differentiated from real masses by
         a. Palpation at physical exam
         b. Sequential change on radiographs
   B. In **late small bowel obstruction,** fluid fills dilated small bowel and appears as tubular soft-tissue masses. The abdomen (bowel) is **devoid of gas ("gasless abdomen")** (see Fig. 6-9).
   C. **Pathologic fluid masses**
      1. **Abscesses**
         a. Soft-tissue mass displacing bowel
         b. May contain mottled gas, or gas within a mass
      2. **Cysts**
         a. Soft-tissue mass.
         b. Renal cysts are most common; also ovarian, splenic, hepatic, choledochal.

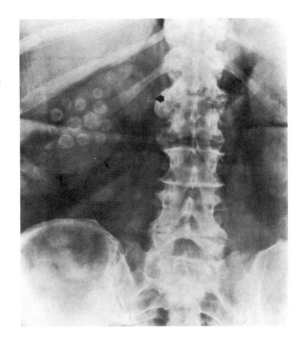

**Fig. 6-19.** *A diameter of greater than 4 mm signifies gallbladder wall thickening (small arrows). The gallbladder wall is not usually seen on plain film. Multiple gallbladder stones are seen in this patient; one stone is seen in the cystic duct (large arrow).*

3. **Pseudocyst**
   a. Pancreatic origin.
   b. Usually found in epigastrium or midabdomen. May occur anywhere in the abdomen (or mediastinum).
   c. Associated pancreatic calcification may aid diagnosis.
   d. Characteristically, anterior gastric (occasionally cephalad) and inferior transverse colonic displacement (Fig. 6-20).

4. **Hematoma, lymphocele, urinoma, and seroma** all may appear as a soft-tissue mass displacing adjacent bowel and other viscera.

D. **Solid masses**
   1. Appear well-defined.
   2. Frequently are palpable.
   3. May have associated speckled calcifications within.
   4. Commonly visualized masses include hypernephroma, uterine leiomyoma, retroperitoneal tumors, pancreatic and gastric carcinoma, nodular liver metastases, ovarian tumors, and bulky bowel carcinoma (Fig. 6-21).
   5. An intrauterine pregnancy, which may have subtle fetal parts, is an important pelvic mass in a young woman (see Fig. 6-36).
   6. Most fluid-filled masses and solid soft-tissue masses cannot be differentiated on plain films; they are the same density except for some fat-containing tumors.

IV. **Calcifications**
   A. Views to aid localization

**Fig. 6-20.** *Pancreatic calcification. Characteristic punctate pancreatic calcifications are seen to the left of the midline in this patient with chronic pancreatitis and a pseudocyst. The transverse colon is displaced inferiorly.*

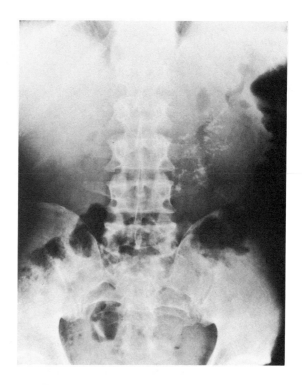

1. Oblique views help differentiate gallbladder stones (anterior), renal calculi (posterior), and costal cartilage calcifications (superficial).
2. Lateral films are helpful for aortic aneurysm calcification.

B. **Clinically nonsignificant calcifications** (Fig. 6-22)

1. **Pelvic phleboliths**
   a. Represent pelvic vein calcifications
   b. Common in adults
   c. Characteristics
      (1) **Location.** Pelvis, usually below the ischial spines
      (2) **Appearance.** Lucent center with thick calcific rim
      (3) **Number.** Often multiple

2. **Mesenteric lymph nodes.** From remote infections or old granulomatous disease
   a. **Location.** Usually mid or low abdomen
   b. **Appearance.** Clumpy, amorphous, may be larger than 1 cm
   c. **Number.** One or several

3. **Nonaneurysmal arterial calcification**
   a. Most frequently in the aorta, or in iliac, splenic, or renal arteries.
   b. Occasionally significant for ischemic symptoms.
   c. Generally not relevant for the patient with abdominal pain in the emergency room.
   d. When the artery is **focally dilated,** it is considered

**Fig. 6-21.** *Solid masses usually are well defined and will displace bowel. Small bowel is displaced from the pelvis on the plain film (**A**), and the sigmoid colon is displaced on the barium enema (**B**). CT, MRI, or ultrasound best determines the origin of these masses, although size alone suggests ovarian as most likely (which this was). The rounded pelvic calcifications are characteristic of phleboliths.*

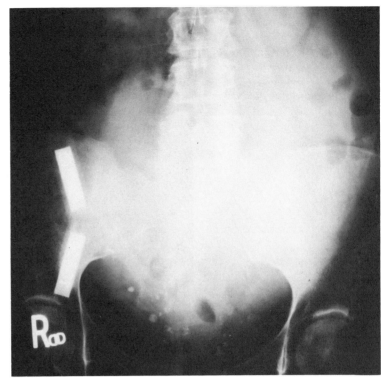

A

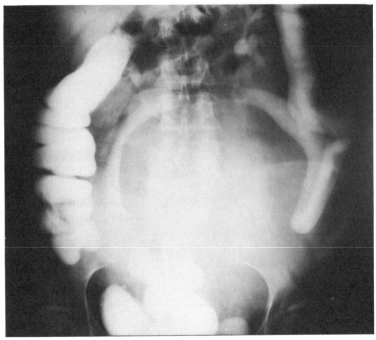

B

**Fig. 6-22.** *Various types of calcifications are seen in this patient. GS = gallstones; CC = costal cartilage; LN = mesenteric lymph node; upper arrows = left common iliac artery; PH = phleboliths; lower arrows = vas deferens.*

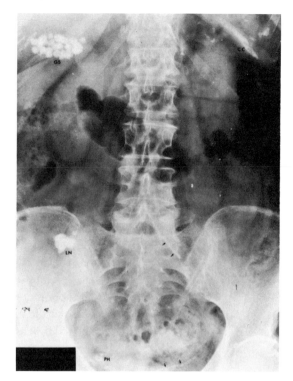

significant (although not necessarily relevant to the current abdominal problem).

    **e.** Arterial calcifications in a young patient usually signify diabetes or hyperlipidemia.

  **4. Granulomata** in the spleen or liver

    **a. Source.** From healed histoplasmosis or tuberculosis

    **b. Appearance.** Few or multiple small punctate calcifications

  **5. Costal cartilage calcifications**

    **a.** Frequently found in middle-aged or elderly patients.

    **b.** Usually symmetric and frequently extensive.

    **c.** Oblique views confirm their anterior superficial position.

**C. Significant calcifications**

  **1. Gallbladder stones.** Twenty percent are opaque and visible (see Fig. 6-19).

    **a. Appearance.** Faceted, occasionally only the rim may be calcified.

    **b. Site.** Right upper quadrant, right midabdomen.

    **c. Number.** One or many.

    **d.** Migration and atypical sites of gallstones

      **(1)** Common bile duct

      **(2)** Cystic duct (see Fig. 6-19)

      **(3)** Small bowel (gallstone ileus)

**e. Ultrasound** is the technique of choice for evaluating the biliary system.

**2. Gallbladder wall calcification**

　　**a.** "Porcelain gallbladder"

　　**b.** Increased incidence of gallbladder carcinoma

**3. Renal stones.** Most are visible because of calcification (80%).

　　**a. Appearance.** Dense (calcium phosphate) or faint (cystine)

　　**b. Site.** Within the kidney

　　　　**(1) Nephrolithiasis.** Stones in the collecting system

　　　　**(2) Nephrocalcinosis.** Punctate or tubular calcifications within the parenchyma

　　**c. Size.** Varies from a few millimeters to staghorn

　　**d.** Ureteral stones

　　　　**(1)** May be quite small

　　　　**(2)** Must be meticulously searched for along the course of the ureters (see Fig. 6-23)

　　　　**(3)** May occur in association with renal stones or may represent a fragment of the original stone

**4. Aneurysmal arterial calcifications** (Fig. 6-24)

　　**a. Aorta is most frequent;** also in iliac, renal, splenic, and hepatic arteries.

　　**b. Appearance.** Linear or curvilinear; one or both walls may be seen.

　　**c. Site.** Convex laterally to the left of the lumbar spine.

　　**d.** Diagnostic films. **Lateral and AP abdominal film.**

　　**e.** The absence of calcium does not include or exclude aneurysm.

　　**f.** Ultrasound is the procedure of choice for evaluating for aneurysm.

　　**g.** Unilateral absence of psoas may occur with leak from an aortic aneurysm.

**5. Calcification in benign masses** (Fig. 6-25A)

　　**a. Causes.** Old abscess; hematoma; pancreatic pseudocyst; renal, hepatic, or echinococcal cyst; mucocele.

　　**b. Appearance.** Curvilinear = cyst; clumpy = old abscess or hematoma.

　　**c.** Uterine calcification

　　　　**(1)** Irregular and amorphous

　　　　**(2)** Leiomyoma or leiomyosarcoma (indistinguishable)

　　**d.** Calcification or ossification of fetal skeletal parts. Careful scrutiny is crucial to avoid further radiation to an unborn fetus (see Fig. 6-36).

**6. Calcification in malignant mass** (Fig. 6-25B)

　　**a.** Irregular, amorphous calcifications (e.g., hypernephroma, ovarian carcinoma, hepatoma)

**Fig. 6-23.** *Differentiating pelvic calcifications.* **A.** *Three phleboliths are seen on the right (long arrows). The upper two have dense rims and central lucencies, pathognomonic of phleboliths. The left calcification (short arrow) is more homogeneously calcified; it could either be a phlebolith or a ureteral stone.* **B.** *The intravenous urogram shows the left calcification to be an obstructing ureteral stone (white arrow). This high-grade obstruction caused rupture of the intrarenal collecting system, resulting in extravasation and retroperitoneal dissection of contrast (black arrow).*

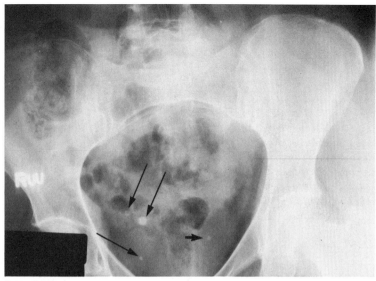

A

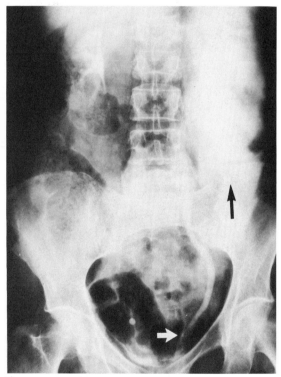

B

**Fig. 6-24.** *Calcified abdominal aortic aneurysm. **A.** The supine film shows a huge mass with a calcified wall (arrows) displacing the colon. Most aortic aneurysms are smaller and are difficult to see if the calcified wall overlies the spine. **B.** The lateral abdominal view is better than the supine film for visualizing smaller aortic aneurysm calcifications (arrows). Ultrasound is more sensitive than plain radiographs and calcification is unnecessary for visualization.*

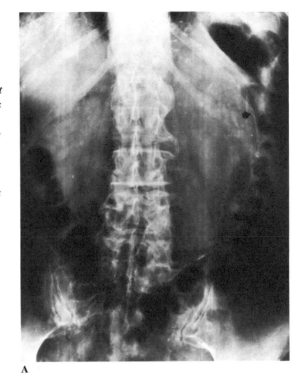

A

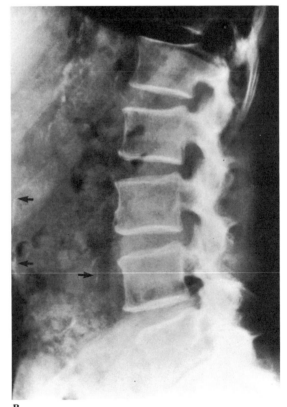

B

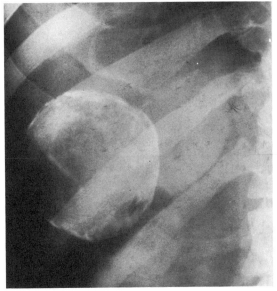

**Fig. 6-25.** *Intrahepatic calcifications. The smoothly rounded peripheral calcification in patient A is characteristic of an echinococcal cyst in the liver. Patient B has irregular calcifications clustered in the liver (arrows). Such an appearance signifies a tumor, in this instance, hepatoma.*

A

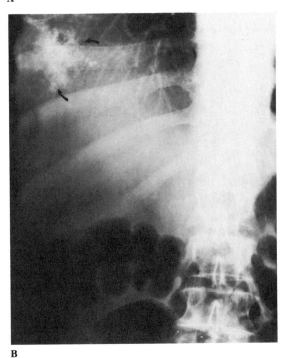

B

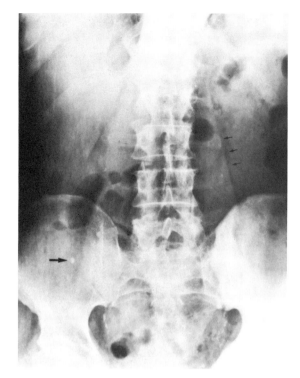

**Fig. 6-26.** *Appendiocolith. The location of an appendicolith (single arrow) is quite variable. This patient has none of the secondary signs of appendicitis except for focal ileus. Note that the psoas margins are distinct (small arrows) and the scoliosis present is convex towards the appendix (opposite of appendicitis). A finding of scoliosis away from the inflamed side may be helpful but is nonspecific.*

      **b.** Mucinous adenocarcinomas
        **(1)** Small punctate calcifications.
        **(2) Causes.** Gastric, colonic, ovarian, or pancreatic tumors
        **(3)** Primary or metastatic lesions
    **7. Appendicoliths** ( Fig. 6-26 )
    **8. Caveat.** Densities confused for calcium include residual barium, foreign bodies, and retained lymphangiographic or myelographic contrast material

**V. Stripes**
  **A. Psoas stripe** ( Fig. 6-26 )
    **1.** Lucency along the lateral margin of the psoas muscle
    **2.** Created by posterior pararenal fat along the lateral margin of the psoas
    **3.** Nonvisualization
      **a.** Occurs in 20 percent of normal people
      **b.** Scoliosis
      **c.** Pathologic nonvisualization
        **(1)** Inflammation (pancreatitis, peri- or pararenal abscess, psoas abscess)
        **(2)** Tumor
        **(3)** Blood (retroperitoneal hematoma)
  **B. Properitoneal fat and flank stripe** (see Fig. 6-47)
    **1.** Lateral and circumferential extension of posterior pararenal fat.

2. Properitoneal fat is lucent; the width is variable, larger with obese patients.

3. **Focal or unilateral absence** implies adjacent inflammation (e.g., appendicitis with periappendiceal abscess).

4. Used as a sensitive indicator of *ascites*—thick flanked stripe.

   a. The space between the properitoneal fat stripe and the lateral wall of the ascending or descending colon is a potential peritoneal space (paracolic gutter).

   b. Small amounts of ascites or blood accumulate and widen the distance between the flank stripe and the colon.

   c. **Caveat.** Fluid-filled small bowel may normally occupy the paracolic gutter and give a false impression of ascites.

VI. **Lungs**

   A. The lung bases frequently are easily seen, especially with a bright light on abdominal x-rays.

   B. Check for unsuspected pneumonia, nodules, pleural effusions, or pneumothorax (Fig. 6-27).

VII. **Bones.** Abdominal radiograph occasionally is helpful and should be perused in the emergency room setting.

   A. **Scoliosis** may indicate inflammation (concave toward the inflamed side).

   B. **Trauma.** Examine carefully for fractures; may help pinpoint a traumatized adjacent organ (e.g., left lower ribs associated with splenic injury or transverse processes of midlumbar vertebra associated with renal injury).

   C. **Tumor.** Destruction of vertebral pedicles or ribs, lucent or blastic pelvic bones or vertebrae.

SPECIFIC ORGAN AND COMPARTMENTAL DISEASES

I. **Right upper quadrant**

   A. **Gallbladder**

      1. **Cholecystitis.** Acute and chronic cholecystitis may have no plain film findings; however, suggestive or diagnostic findings include:

         a. Emphysematous cholecystitis

            (1) Abnormal **gas** in the **wall or lumen** of the gallbladder or in the **pericholecystic tissues**

            (2) Most frequently seen in **diabetics** with *Escherichia coli* (see Figs. 6-13 and 6-14).

         b. May see gallstones or cystic duct stones or both (see Fig. 6-19)

         c. Associated gas in the biliary tree with gas-forming organisms (see Fig. 6-12)

**Fig. 6-27.** *Pneumothorax best seen on abdominal radiographs. The supine view of the left upper quadrant in patient **A** demonstrates a pneumothorax. Air is seen above the diaphragm adjacent to the diseased lung. The anterior pleural reflection is also seen sloping obliquely upward (arrows), outlined by the air of the pneumothorax. The anterior pleural reflection is not seen normally. The anterior pleural reflection is differentiated from the posterior pleural reflection seen in patient **B** by its oblique orientation. The posterior pleural reflection is seen in normal patients and is oriented more horizontally (arrows).*

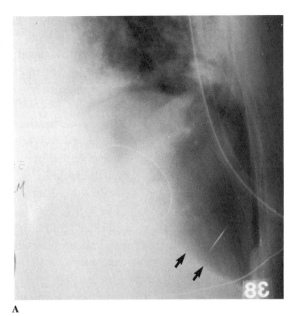

A

B

    **d.** Localized right upper quadrant ileus

2. **Hydrops** (see Fig. 6-19)
       **a.** Previously mentioned findings of cholecystitis may or may not be present.
       **b.** Right upper quadrant soft-tissue mass representing the enlarged gallbladder

3. **Cholangitis**
       **a.** May see gallstones, cystic duct stones, or common duct stones.
       **b.** Gas-forming organisms may produce intra- or extra-hepatic bile duct gas.

4. **Gallstone ileus**
       **a. Mechanical small bowel obstruction from a gallstone** that has eroded into the gastrointestinal tract
       **b.** Most frequent in elderly females (see Fig. 6-12)
       **c.** Radiographic findings

       **(1) Gas** in the biliary tree from the enteric fistula (cholecystoduodenal most frequent)

       **(2) Small bowel obstruction** (partial or complete)

       **(3)** May see remaining *gallstones* within the gallbladder

       **(4)** Offending distal **gallstone causing obstruction in the small intestine** (most commonly at the ileocecal valve)

**B. Liver**

  **1. Hepatic abscess** (see Fig. 6-15)

    **a. Gas** within the liver; may be mottled, usually irregular.

    **b.** There may be generalized hepatomegaly or protrusion of a lobe of the liver or the liver may be of normal size and configuration.

    **c.** Upright film may show **air-fluid level** within the cavity.

    **d.** Associated right pleural effusion or basilar atelectasis.

  **2. Echinococcus cyst** (see Fig. 6-25A). Rounded, curvilinear intrahepatic calcification

  **3. Alcoholic liver disease**

    **a. Variable-sized.** Hepatomegaly with fatty infiltration, or small liver with cirrhosis

    **b.** Associated ascites and splenomegaly with portal venous hypertension

  **4. Hepatitis**

    **a.** No specific findings, other than possible hepatic enlargement with acute hepatitis

    **b.** Liver may be small with severe chronic active hepatitis and fibrosis.

  **5. Hepatic tumors**

    **a.** Generalized hepatomegaly or focal enlargement

    **b.** Types

      **(1)** *Hepatoma.* Twenty percent contain amorphous calcification (see Fig. 6-25B).

      **(2) Metastatic disease.** Punctate calcifications seen with mucinous adenocarcinoma from gastrointestinal tract, pancreas, or ovary.

    **c. Focal nodular hyperplasia and hepatic adenoma.** May present as chronic pain and a right upper quadrant mass or as an acute abdomen with marked right upper quadrant pain and tenderness in a woman of childbearing age taking birth control pills.

      **(1)** Generalized hepatomegaly or focal liver mass in the right upper quadrant.

      **(2)** May see hemoperitoneum if the tumor ruptures and bleeds (adenoma bleeds more commonly) (see Fig. 6-47).

**Fig. 6-28.** *Gastric outlet obstruction. The stomach is markedly dilated in this patient with acute duodenal obstruction due to peptic disease.*

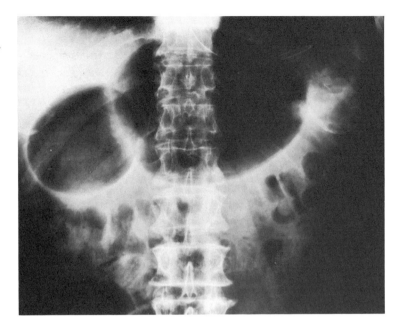

       **d. Hemangioma**

         **(1)** Most common benign hepatic tumor

         **(2)** Occasionally spokelike or rounded calcification

    **C. Subphrenic and subhepatic abscesses.** These occur most frequently postoperatively or associated with perforated duodenal ulcer, ruptured appendiceal abscess, or gangrenous cholecystitis.

       **1.** Abnormal extraintestinal gas above or below the liver (see Fig. 6-15).

       **2.** May have an **air-fluid level** on upright or decubitus film.

       **3.** With a left subphrenic abscess, the stomach may be displaced inferiorly and separated from the hemidiaphragm.

       **4.** Elevated ipsilateral hemidiaphragm.

       **5.** Associated ipsilateral pleural effusion.

    **D. Obstructive jaundice**

       **1.** Usually no plain film findings.

       **2.** Two radiographic abnormalities may occur: (a) common bile duct stone and (b) right-sided soft-tissue mass—pancreatic (carcinoma, pseudocyst), gallbladder carcinoma, adenopathy, or Courvoisier gallbladder.

**II. Epigastrium and left upper quadrant**

  **A. Stomach and duodenum**

    **1. Peptic ulcer disease.** The **complications** are visible radiographically.

      **a. Perforation.** Free intraperitoneal, lesser sac, or confined retroperitoneal gas (streaks) (see Fig. 6-1). (Absence of free air does not exclude perforation.)

**b. Penetration.** Posterior duodenal ulcer can penetrate the pancreas and cause signs of pancreatitis.

**c. Gastric outlet obstruction**

(1) From acute ulcer disease with intense edema or chronic disease with scarring.

(2) Stomach is markedly dilated (Fig. 6-28).

**d. Bleeding**

(1) Upper abdominal or diffuse ileus

(2) Often no radiographic signs

**2. Gastritis.** Focal epigastric or upper abdominal ileus may be seen.

**3. Gastroenteritis**

a. Mild dilatation and possible air-fluid levels in the small bowel and, less frequently, large bowel.

b. This pattern is similar to that of aerophagia.

**B. Spleen.** Splenic abscess, infarct

1. Splenic enlargement or left upper quadrant mass

2. Focal ileus, left pleural effusion

3. Occurs with underlying sepsis, endocarditis, immunosuppression (abscess)

**III. Right lower quadrant**

**A. Appendicitis.** Abnormal plain film findings are seen in about 50 percent of instances.

1. The most **diagnostic** finding is a calcified right lower quadrant **appendicolith** (8–10%); calcifications frequently are faint or overlie bony structures (see Fig. 6-26).

2. Abnormal **gas patterns**

a. Focal right lower quadrant ileus most common.

b. Diffuse ileus.

c. Cecal air-fluid level may occur.

3. **Small bowel obstruction** is uncommon.

4. **Free air** is **rare.**

5. Several nonspecific findings of inflammatory disease may be seen (Fig. 6-29)

a. **Scoliosis,** concave toward right lower quadrant.

b. **Lower psoas margin obliteration**

c. **Obliteration** of the adjacent **properitoneal fat stripe** from the adjacent inflammation

6. **Periappendiceal abscess.** Findings similar to appendicitis (Figs. 6-30 and 6-31)

a. Right lower quadrant soft-tissue **mass**

b. **Mottled gas** in the abscess

c. Adjacent displacement of **bowel gas**

**B. Regional enteritis** (Crohn's disease). Radiographic findings usually in the right lower quadrant, although any of

**Fig. 6-29.** *Appendicitis and peri-appendiceal abscess. This patient has an appendicolith, scoliosis convex toward the left, poor definition of the right psoas margin, a bubbly collection of gas to the right of the fourth lumbar vertebra, and medial displacement of the ascending colon.*

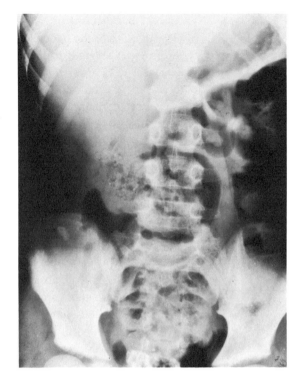

**Fig. 6-30.** *Periappendiceal abscess. There is a right lower quadrant mass (arrows) but no appendicolith. Abundant mildly dilated small bowel gas suggests a diffuse ileus or early small bowel obstruction.*

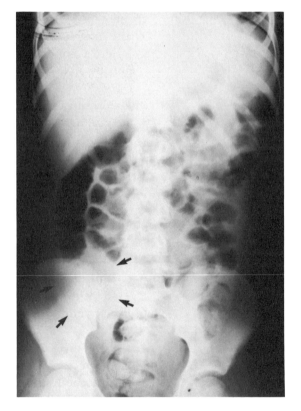

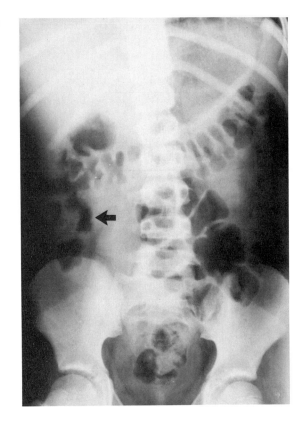

**Fig. 6-31.** *The wall of the cecum and ascending colon is thickened and edematous (arrow) in response to a perforated appendix. The midportion of the right psoas stripe is obliterated and the scoliosis is concave to the right.*

the small bowel and most of the colon can be involved (Fig. 6-32).

1. **Mucosal and submucosal thickening, fixed loops** of small bowel
2. Focal **ileus**
3. Soft-tissue **mass** with possible abscess
4. May present as **small bowel obstruction**
5. Associated findings
   a. Renal stones (usually oxalate)
   b. Gallstones
   c. Sacroiliitis with sacroiliac joint sclerosis (associated with positive HLA $B_{27}$ antigen)

C. **Meckel's diverticulum**
   1. Nonspecific inflammatory findings mimic appendicitis—right lower quadrant ileus and scoliosis.
   2. May present as small bowel obstruction.
   3. Calcification may occur within the diverticulum.
   4. Radionuclide scan is the diagnostic procedure of choice with bleeding.

IV. **Left lower quadrant**
   A. **Diverticulitis** (Fig. 6-33)
      1. Left lower quadrant or pelvic soft-tissue mass (abscess or phlegmon).

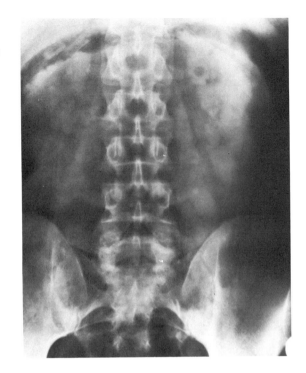

**Fig. 6-32.** *In regional enteritis, or Crohn's disease, small and/or large bowel may be involved. In this patient, the colon is inflamed and edematous. The sacroiliac joints also are sclerotic (the associated sacroiliitis).*

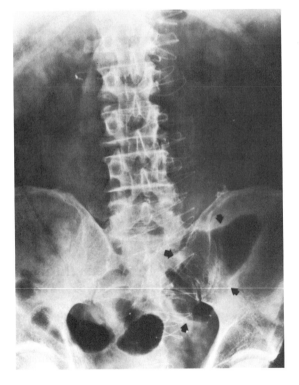

**Fig. 6-33.** *Diverticular abscess. Note the large extraluminal gas collection in the left lower quadrant (arrows) (see Fig. 5-16).*

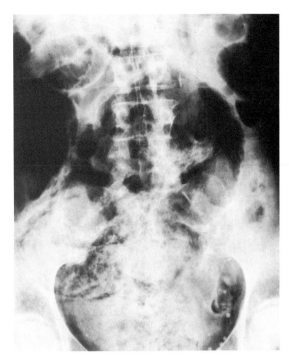

2. Bubbly extraluminal gas is diagnostic of abscess.
3. Abnormal bowel gas patterns
   a. Localized left lower quadrant ileus
   b. Large bowel obstruction
4. Free air is rare.

**B. Left-sided colonic carcinoma,** including splenic flexure and descending and sigmoid colon (see Fig. 6-8)
1. Partial or complete large bowel obstruction.
2. Lesion may be visible as irregular mass at the distal aspect of the distended large intestine.

**V. Pelvis**

**A. Rectum**

**1. Fecal impaction**

a. **Clinical setting.** Elderly patients on antiparkinsonian medications or patients with altered electrolytes (hypokalemia, hypocalcemia) (Fig. 6-34)

b. Radiographic signs
   (1) Copious, irregular, bubbly fecal material within the confines of a dilated rectum and sigmoid
   (2) Excessive stool throughout much of the left and often the right colon

c. May have partial large bowel obstruction

d. Occurs in younger patients as "psychogenic colon" (different from aganglionosis in Hirschsprung's disease)

**Fig. 6-35.** *"Straight lines should be viewed with suspicion," as in this patient with a broom handle in the rectosigmoid colon (arrows). While there is no extraluminal gas to suggest perforation, its absence does not exclude perforation.*

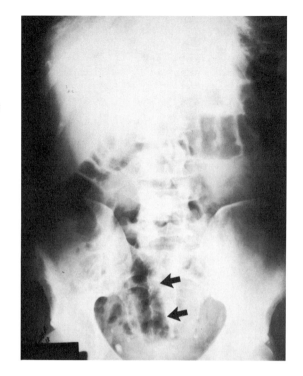

**Fig. 6-36.** *Denied pregnancy. Fetal ribs (arrows) are seen overlying the right side of the sacrum in this patient who had an intravenous urogram. The dome of the contrast-filled bladder is indented by the gravid uterus.*

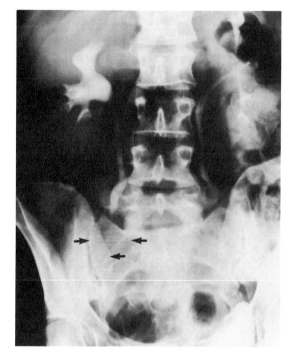

    **e. Caveat.** Barium enema indicated to rule out occult **obstructing carcinoma.**

  2. **Foreign bodies.** Particularly in the male homosexual population, an assortment of items (bottles, vibrators, needles, handles) may be seen (Fig. 6-35).

    **a.** These may cause rectal perforation, which results in retroperitoneal gas (see Fig. 6-4) and, possibly, abscess formation.

    **b.** Lateral film and Gastrografin enema may be necessary to ascertain whether perforation has occurred.

  3. **Rectal carcinoma.** Findings of large bowel obstruction or ileus

**B. Gynecologic entities** (best investigated with ultrasound initially)

  1. **Tuboovarian abscess** (TOA):

    **a.** Soft-tissue pelvic mass.

    **b.** May be gas within the mass.

    **c.** Mass effect with bowel displacement and indentation on the bladder.

    **d.** Uterus may be seen as a separate structure.

  2. **Pregnancy.** May be denied, unrealized, or hidden by a teenager in the presence of parents.

    **a.** Early in pregnancy, the skeletal parts may be faint (Fig. 6-36).

    **b.** Ectopic pregnancy may result in a pelvic mass and hemoperitoneum.

  3. **Lost intrauterine device**

    **a.** Opaque intrauterine device (IUD) may be seen eccentrically positioned or outside the confines of the uterus.

    **b.** Ultrasound frequently useful to identify the IUD within or outside the uterus.

  4. **Ovarian tumors** (see Fig. 6-21)

    **a.** Bowel displacement

    **b.** Mass may be very large

    **c.** Faint punctate, amorphous calcifications or teeth (dermoid)

  5. Ultrasound is excellent for further delineation of pelvic masses.

**VI. Retroperitoneum**

**A. Pancreas**

  1. **Acute pancreatitis** (Fig. 6-37)

    **a.** Several indirect and nonspecific findings on adjacent bowel caused by pancreatic inflammation

      **(1)** Focal ileus. "Sentinel loop"

      **(2)** "Colon cutoff." No gas distal to splenic flexure

**Fig.** 6-37. *A. Acute pancreatitis. Calcifications (small arrow) of chronic pancreatitis are present; a sentinel loop of dilated small bowel (large arrows) adjacent to the pancreas is a response to acute inflammation. The bowel wall is edematous, manifested by small bowel wall thickening (plicae should be no thicker than 3 mm normally). B. Another patient with acute pancreatitis demonstrates the "colon cutoff" sign. The transverse colon is dilated up to the splenic flexure (solid arrow) with little colonic gas distally. A small bowel sentinel loop (open arrow) also is present. The plical markings completely transverse the diameter of the bowel, assuring that this loop is small bowel. Colonic haustral markings only partially transverse the diameter of the bowel except in the cecum.*

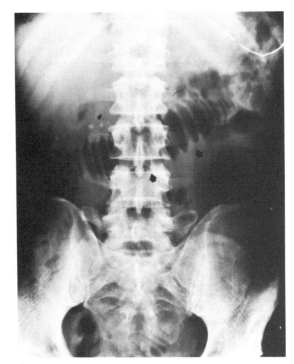

A

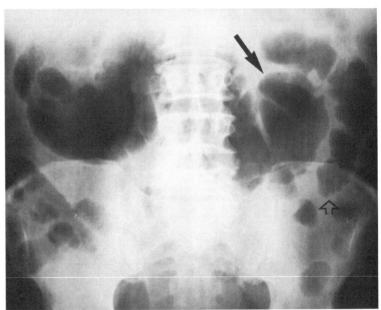

B

**Fig. 6-38.** *Pancreatic abscess. A characteristic mottled and bubbly appearance of an abscess is seen in the pancreatic bed and lesser sac region (arrows). Barium from a prior barium enema outlines the colon. The gas below the diaphragm is in the superiorly displaced stomach.*

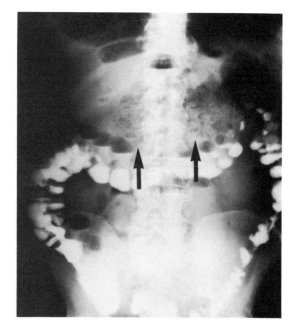

(3) Increased soft-tissue distance (inflammation) between the transverse colon and the stomach

(4) Absent psoas margins caused by retroperitoneal pancreatic fluid dissection

(5) Associated pancreatic calcifications may or may not be present.

**b. Thoracic changes**

(1) **Pleural effusion.** Left side alone, or left side greater than right

(2) Platelike atelectasis at the lung bases (left greater than right)

(3) Pulmonary edema (rare)

**2. Pancreatic pseudocyst** (see Fig. 6-20)

**a. Soft-tissue mass** anywhere in the abdomen or mediastinum

**b.** Commonly, **displacement** of the stomach, usually anteriorly and superiorly

**c.** Transverse colon and small bowel displacement (usually inferiorly)

**d.** Uncommonly, curvilinear calcification in the pseudocyst wall

**3. Pancreatic and lesser sac abscess** (Fig. 6-38)

**a.** A severe complication of acute phlegmonous pancreatitis.

**b.** Findings of acute pancreatitis also may be present.

**c.** Mottled gas and mass in the pancreatic bed, lesser sac, or both.

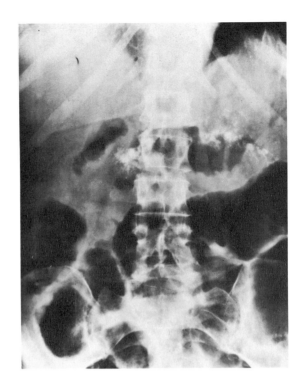

4. **Chronic pancreatitis** (Fig. 6-39)
   a. **Ductal calcifications** in alcoholic pancreatitis
   b. **Multiple** calcifications
   c. Most frequently in the pancreatic **head** (overlies L2 vertebra)

B. **Genitourinary diseases**
   1. **Kidney**
      a. **Pyelonephritis** (Fig. 6-40)
         (1) **Acute pyelonephritis.** May have asymmetric renal enlargement
         (2) **Emphysematous pyelonephritis**
      b. **Renal and perinephric abscess**
         (1) **Staphylococcal and gram-negative organisms are most common.**
         (2) X-ray findings
            (a) Focal renal or perirenal mass
            (b) Ill-defined renal margin
            (c) Obliteration of the psoas (particularly upper portion)
            (d) **Scoliosis** concave toward affected side
            (e) **Gas** in the **renal and perinephric space**
            (f) Fixation of the kidneys caused by inflam-mation—lack of normal excursion of the kidneys on separate inspiratory-expiratory radiographs

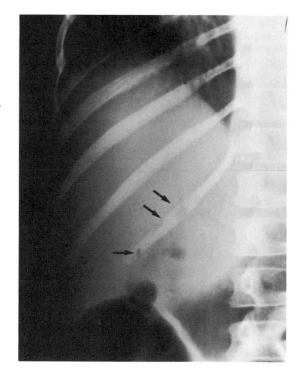

**Fig. 6-40.** *Emphysematous pyelonephritis. There is abnormal gas adjacent to the kidney in this patient (arrows). These thin linear collections of gas inevitably are outside a visceral lumen. A lateral or oblique view would demonstrate the relatively posterior position of the peripheral gas.*

      **c. Renal calculi**
        **(1) Nephrolithiasis** (calculi in the collecting system).
        **(2) Nephrocalcinosis** (calculi in the renal cortex).
        **(3)** Oblique views confirm renal location of stones.
    **2. Ureteral obstruction** (see Fig. 6-23)
      **a. Calculi**
        **(1)** Present as renal colic radiating down the flank into the lower pelvis
        **(2)** Radiographic findings
          **(a) Obstructing stone may be small and faint** along ureteral course; differentiate from phleboliths.
          **(b) Commonest site of obstruction is ureterovesicular junction** (UVJ).
          **(c)** Affected kidney may be enlarged.
          **(d) Intravenous urogram** ensures diagnosis.
      **b.** Tumor
        **(1) "Frozen pelvis"** from primary gynecologic tumor, bladder tumor, drop metastasis (from stomach or pancreatic carcinoma), or lymphoma can cause uni- or bilateral renal obstruction.
        **(2)** Kidneys may be enlarged because of obstruction.
**VII. Specific bowel diseases**
    **A. Large bowel obstruction** (LBO). Etiologies include carcinoma, diverticulitis, fecal impaction, hernia, volvulus,

**Fig. 6-41.** *Cecal volvulus. The hallmark of volvulus or any closed loop obstruction is bowel that is dilated well out of proportion to any other bowel gas. In this patient, the mobile cecum has twisted about its axis (large arrow), is markedly dilated, and lies obliquely across the abdomen up to the left upper quadrant (small arrows).*

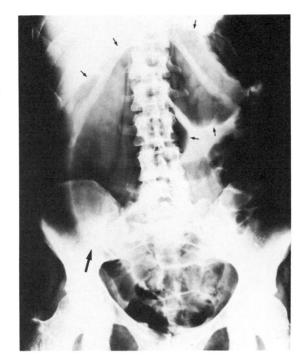

**Fig. 6-42.** *Pathognomonic appearance of sigmoid volvulus. The grossly distended loop of sigmoid fills the middle and right sections of the abdomen. The point at which the loop has twisted on itself is seen (arrow). The tapered "beak-shaped" appearance of the right side of the loop at the point of twisting indicates the characteristic narrowing adjacent to the point of obstruction.*

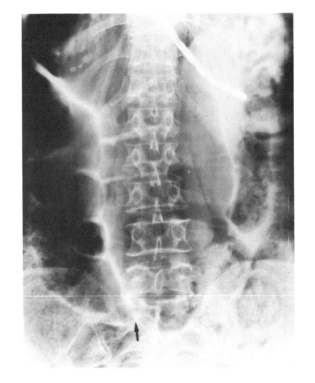

and intussusception (Figs. 6-8, 6-34, 6-41, and 6-42).

1. **Volvulus,** generally of two types—cecal and sigmoid (gastric volvulus is rare)

    a. **Cecal** (Fig. 6-41)

        (1) Form of malrotation—nonfixation of large bowel to the posterior abdominal wall because cecum and ascending colon are on extended mesenteries.

        (2) Findings

            (a) Cecum twists on itself, causing large gas collection (the cecum itself) anywhere in the abdomen, frequently in the left upper quadrant.

            (b) Axis of the cecum (dilated loop) points to the right lower quadrant.

            (c) Associated small bowel dilatation proximal to obstruction.

            (d) Decreased or absent distal colonic gas.

    b. **Sigmoid (Fig. 6-42)**

        (1) Sigmoid twists on its mesentery.

        (2) Closed loop sigmoid obstruction forms, and there is associated proximal colonic dilatation.

        (3) Inverted U from pelvis projecting upward into abdomen is the sigmoid volvulus itself.

2. **Intussusception** (see Fig. 8-15)

    a. Most frequently enterocolic

    b. Lead point from tumor or polyp originating in the distal ileum (in adults)

    c. Often idiopathic in young children

    d. Transverse colon

        (1) Soft-tissue mass representing lead point in right colon

        (2) Proximal large or small bowel obstruction

B. **Closed loop obstruction**

    1. Two points of obstruction in small or large intestine

    2. **Etiology.** Strangulated internal or femoral hernia, volvulus

    3. Bowel infarct and gangrene occur because of ischemia.

    4. Radiographic findings

        a. Inverted gas-filled U loop with effaced folds. If distention is much greater than other bowel gas, a closed loop obstruction is the diagnosis.

        b. On serial follow-up films, the loop is unchanged.

        c. Closed loop may be fluid-filled and appear as a mass.

        d. May be two loops of distended bowel: the closed loop itself and the proximal obstructed bowel.

        e. Thickening of bowel wall signifies edema and vascular compromise.

        f. Microperforation leads to gas in bowel well.

**Table 6-2.** *Sequence of Plain Film Findings in Bowel Ischemia*

| | |
|---|---|
| Early: | Thickening of folds and bowel wall (more than 3 mm in small bowel) |
| | Dilatation of bowel may or may not be seen |
| Later: | Effacement of folds with thickened wall |
| | Thumbprinting |
| | Air in bowel wall |
| Late: | Air in portal venous system |

      **g.** Free air is late and ominous.

**C. Vascular compromise of bowel** (Table 6-2)

    **1.** Spectrum includes ischemia, infarct, and, eventually, gangrene with perforation.

    **2.** Severity depends on collateral vascular flow.

    **3. Mechanisms**

      **a.** Decreased arterial perfusion

      **b.** Arterial embolization

      **c.** Thrombosis of arteries or veins

    **4.** Common **sites** are in the distribution of the superior mesenteric artery (jejunum to splenic flexure).

    **5. Radiographic findings** (Fig. 6-43)

      **a.** Thickened *thumbprinted* loop or loops of small or large intestine (submucosal blood and edema).

      **b. Dilatation** of small and large bowel, either focally or diffusely.

      **c.** Bowel may have a **rigid appearance,** with sequential films showing **fixed,** abnormal loops.

      **d.** Bowel loops abnormally separated by thick walls.

      **e.** Valvulae conniventes are thickened or obliterated.

      **f.** Peritonitis with **ascites** carries a poor prognosis.

      **g. Abnormal gas**

        **(1) Gas in the bowel wall** signifies microperforation.

        **(2) Portal venous gas** heralds death in most patients (see Fig. 6-11).

      **h.** Radiographic findings are the same whatever the cause.

**D. Inflammatory bowel disease**

    **1.** Regional enteritis. Findings include (see Fig. 6-32)

      **a.** Small bowel obstruction

      **b.** Mass effect

      **c.** Abscess

      **d.** Thickened fixed bowel loops

      **e.** Right lower quadrant findings (most frequent)

    **2.** Ulcerative colitis (Fig. 6-44)

      **a.** Toxic megacolon

      **b.** Thickened large bowel

      **c.** Thumbprinting

**E. Toxic megacolon** (Fig. 6-45)

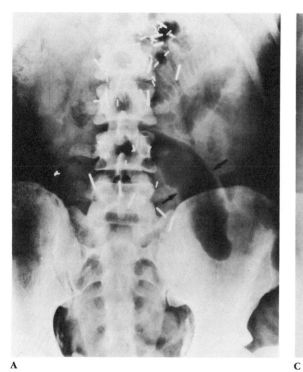

A

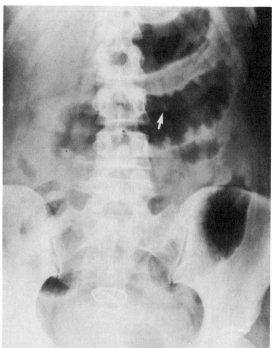

C

**Fig. 6-43.** *Mesenteric ischemia. These three patients demonstrate the findings of edematous bowel caused by ischemia. In patient A, an amorphous loop of small bowel has a thickened wall and no normal plical markings (arrows). This is a strangulated closed loop obstruction. Patient B (arrows) shows "thumbprinting" of the bowel wall, as does patient C. "Thumbprints" represent edematous folds or intramural bleeding (arrow).*

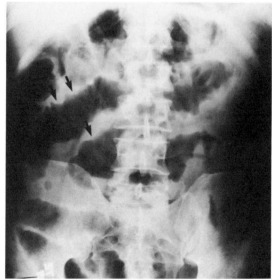

B

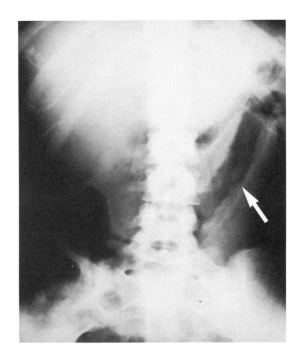

**Fig. 6-44.** *Ulcerative colitis. The colon is edematous and haustral markings are obliterated. Mounds of edematous mucosa are visible (arrow); with advanced disease, the colon becomes narrowed and tubular in appearance.*

**Fig. 6-45.** *Toxic megacolon presents as markedly dilated colon. The transverse colon frequently is most dilated because of its nondependent position. Haustral markings are effaced, and the colon may appear edematous.*

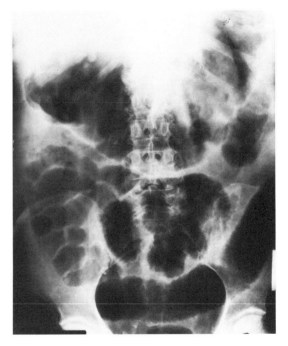

**Fig. 6-46.** *In massive ascites, there is a haziness throughout the abdomen. Gas within small bowel floats centrally as in this patient. Fluid collecting in the pelvis is seen above the bladder (arrows).*

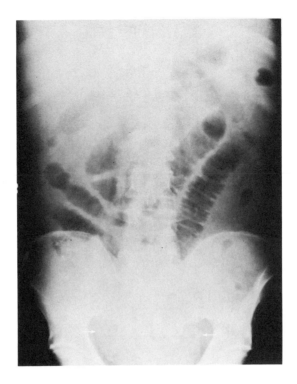

1. Seen with any form of colitis (ulcerative, pseudomembranous, amebic, bacterial).
2. Associated thickened transverse colon.
3. Imminent risk of perforation.
4. **Caveat.** Barium enema is contraindicated in these cases because of risk of perforation.

**VIII. Ascites.** Serous ascitic fluid, exudative peritonitis, hemoperitoneum, or any other diffuse free-flowing intraabdominal fluid may be visible, but they cannot be differentiated by plain film.

**A.** Late and obvious radiographic signs include (Fig. 6-46)

1. Diffuse abdominal haziness
2. Central floating small bowel loops
3. Bulging flanks
4. Separation of bowel loops by fluid

**B. Earlier** and more **subtle findings** may be seen radiographically **before** clinical signs are apparent. These findings include (Fig. 6-47)

1. **Nonvisualization of hepatic and splenic outlines** (caused by fluid floating the organs away from adjacent retroperitoneal and flank fat).
2. Medial displacement of the ascending or descending colon from the lateral abdominal wall by interposed fluid in the paracolic gutter.

**Fig. 6-47.** *Subtle ascites or hemoperitoneum.* **A.** *The flank stripe, which is the density between the colon and properitoneal fat, is only a few millimeters wide normally (arrows).* **B.** *Even small amounts of ascites or hemoperitoneum in the paracolic gutter cause widening (arrows) of the flank stripe.*

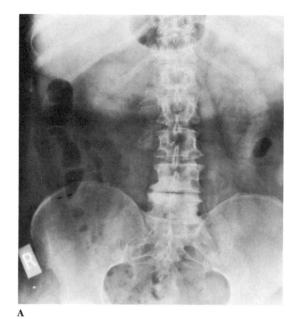

A

B

**Caveat.** The finding is not absolutely specific, as fluid-filled small bowel in the paracolic gutter or collapsed colon may give a similar appearance.

3. "Dog ears," or dependent pelvic fluid in the paravesicular fossae adjacent to the bladder.

SELECTED READINGS

Bundrick TJ, Cho S-R, Brewer WH, Beachley MC. Ascites: Comparison of plain film radiographs with ultrasonograms. Radiology 152:503, 1984.

Cherian MJ, Kumar EN, Cherian K, et al. Prone films of abdomen—a diagnostic tool in intestinal obstruction in children. Radiology 150:613, 1984.

Johnson CD, Rice RP. Acute abdomen: Plain radiographic evaluation. Radiographics 5:259, 1985.

Kelvin FM, Rice RR. Radiologic evaluation of acute abdominal pain arising from the alimentary tract. Radiol Clin North Am 16:25, 1978.

Loughran CF. Review of the plain abdominal radiograph in acute rupture of abdominal aortic aneurysms. Clin Radiol 37:383, 1986.

McCort JJ. Intraperitoneal and retroperitoneal hemorrhage. Radiol Clin North Am 14:391, 1976.

Mirvis SE, Young JWR, Keramati B, et al. Plain film evaluation of patients with abdominal pain: Are three radiographs necessary? AJR 147:501, 1986.

Williams SM, Harned RK, Hultman SA, Quaife MA. Psoas sign: Reevaluation. Radiographics 5:525, 1985.

# 7 Thoracoabdominal Trauma

*Eric vanSonnenberg and James T. Rhea*

The effects of thoracic trauma range from mild soft-tissue contusion to sudden death from aortic transection. Early radiographic recognition of the effects of trauma and proper x-ray interpretation frequently are pivotal to the patient's outcome. Effects of therapy and resuscitative devices must be assessed radiographically to ensure optimal functioning. Incorrect positioning of these devices (chest and endotracheal tubes, subclavian catheter, Swan-Ganz catheter, and pacer lines) may be deleterious and must be recognized immediately and corrected.

Motor vehicle accidents are the most common cause of thoracic trauma. It is estimated that over half of vehicular deaths in the United States are caused by chest injuries. While blunt injury is most frequent and most ominous, penetrating wounds to vital structures may be catastrophic as well. Blast injuries with flying missiles also are exceedingly dangerous.

This section will deal with the most common and important chest injuries. Structures and specific abnormalities to check for on x-rays of patients with chest trauma include:

| | |
|---|---|
| Lungs | Pulmonary contusion, hematoma, and atelectasis |
| Pleura | Pneumothorax, hemothorax, or a combination |
| Airways | Signs of bronchial rupture |
| Aorta | Signs of aortic tear |
| Bones | Rib, scapular, sternal, and clavicular fractures |
| Heart | Myocardial or pericardial injury |
| Mediastinum | Esophageal disruption |

CHEST TRAUMA

## I. Lung injuries

### A. Contusion (Fig. 7-1)

1. Usually occurs on the side of the injury, but may occur contralaterally (contra-coup effect).
2. Because of edema, with or without blood leakage into interstitial and alveolar tissues.
3. Radiographic appearance is **patchy consolidation.**
4. Occurs within **4 to 6 hours** of injury.

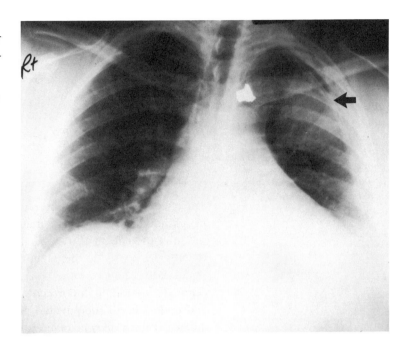

**Fig. 7-1.** *Traumatic pulmonary contusion presents as an area of air-space consolidation with unsharp margins. The contusion (arrow) was caused by a bullet that is projected over the medial aspect of the left clavicle.*

5. Typically, marked improvement within 48 hours and clearing by 1 week (persistence indicates pneumonia).

6. Symptoms and signs vary from relatively asymptomatic to hemoptysis and fever.

B. **Laceration with resultant traumatic cyst or hematoma** (Fig. 7-2)

1. Usually occurs from shearing of lung parenchyma (blunt or blast injuries).

2. Cystic space with hematoma may form.

3. Cyst may be more apparent when blood is expectorated.

4. May persist for weeks to months.

5. Usually resolves spontaneously.

6. Hematoma may appear nodular and resemble tumor.

7. **Penetrating injuries** cause an elongate, cylindrical hematoma, which may persist for weeks.

C. **Atelectasis** (Figs. 7-2 and 7-3)

1. Traumatic mechanisms of atelectasis include:

   a. Bronchial compression by extrinsic hematoma

   b. Bronchial obstruction from blood or mucus

   c. Postcontusion decreased surfactant

   d. Bronchial rupture

   e. Splinting caused by pain

2. Radiographic signs are similar to those of nontraumatic atelectasis.

II. **Bronchial fracture**

A. Most frequent cause is sudden severe compression of the anterior chest wall on the steering wheel of a car.

**Fig. 7-2.** *Hemothorax caused by a stab wound.* **A.** *There is atelectasis of the adjacent lung, suggested by the air bronchograms (branching linear lucent structures) seen through the dense right hemothorax (arrows).* **B.** *A hematoma eventually developed (arrows). The hematoma has sharp margins separating it from adjacent lung. Air within the hematoma suggests an associated bronchial tear.*

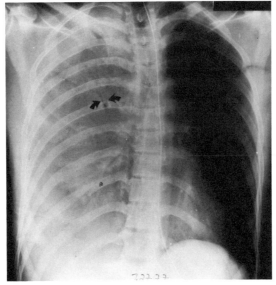

A

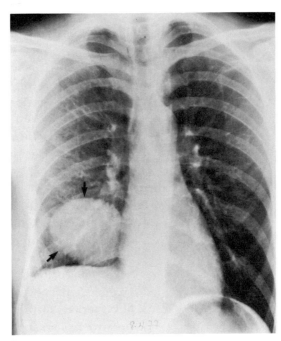

B

**Fig. 7-3.** *Subsegmental platelike atelectasis (arrow) because of pain from trauma and splinting. Platelike atelectasis and scarring look similar on chest x-ray. On subsequent films, however, atelectasis will resolve.*

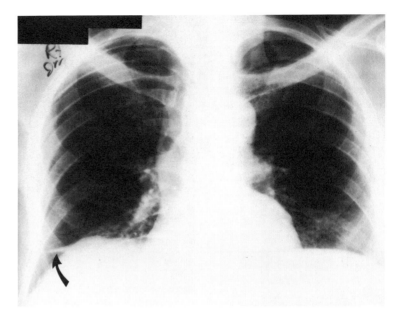

B. **Site** of injury is usually **main stem bronchi,** 1 to 2 cm distal to carina.

C. **Associated injuries** include fracture of first three ribs.

D. **Radiographic findings**

    1. Posttraumatic **tension pneumothorax, unresponsive** to aspiration or chest tube insertion (Fig. 5-12)

    2. **Pneumomediastinum** with or without **subcutaneous emphysema** (Fig. 5-13)

    3. **Atelectasis**

**III. Pleural injuries**

  **A. Pneumothorax**

    1. **Open or closed, tension or simple** pneumothorax; open and tension types are more life-threatening; open must be converted to closed, and tension must be relieved immediately.

    2. Frequently, but not always, associated with **rib fractures.**

    3. More serious in patients with underlying chronic obstructive pulmonary disease (COPD) or heart disease.

    4. **Tension pneumothorax** requires urgent decompression because it compresses normal lung and intrathoracic veins, which leads to decreased venous return and decreased cardiac output.

    5. **Radiographic findings** (Fig. 7-4)

      a. The **key** to pneumothorax visualization is demonstration of the **medially displaced visceral pleural line.**

      b. Increased lucency is seen in the hemithorax peripherally (these findings may be mimicked by skin folds).

**Fig. 7-4.** *Pneumothoraces and pitfalls on chest x-ray.* **A.** *Bilateral pneumothoraces are well seen (arrows). The dense white line represents the visceral pleura. The visceral pleura is displaced inward by the pneumothorax and is sharply marginated. Characteristic findings of pneumothorax are well seen—marked lucency and no bronchovascular lung markings.* **B.** *The small left pneumothorax is difficult to detect in this patient. The only findings are the thin white line representing the visceral pleura (tip of white arrows) and peripheral lucency. This patient also had a contusion at the right base. In addition, there were fractures of the right scapula and ribs (not seen in this film). Osseous abnormalities are best seen by specific bone technique radiographs.* **C.** *A skinfold projects over the lung and is a pitfall for pneumothorax (arrow). Characteristic findings of a skinfold are seen. Note that there is no thin white line representing the visceral pleura; rather, there is a curvilinear change in density. Instead of the sharp visceral pleura line, there is increased density that gradually tapers to the normal lucency of the lung medially. Pulmonary vessels are seen peripheral to the change in density; this helps identify skinfold rather than pneumothorax. The most reliable way to differentiate a pneumothorax from skinfold is to evaluate the margins of the abnormality as above. If there is doubt, obtain an expiration film; a pneumothorax will be much more apparent.*

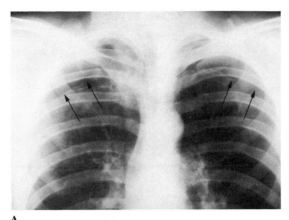

A

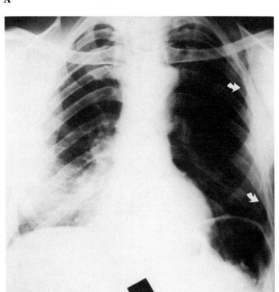

B

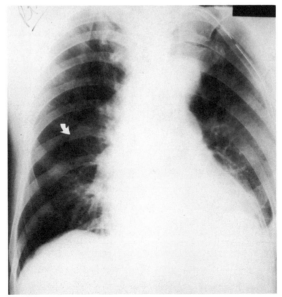

C

c. Pulmonary vessels are absent in the suspected lucent area.

d. Upright **end-expiratory** film shows the pneumothorax to best advantage; the unchanged size of the pneumothorax in expiration occupies relatively more of the hemithorax than in inspiration, and hence it is easier to visualize.

e. In bedridden patients, **cross-table lateral or lateral decubitus films** may lead to diagnosis if the anteroposterior (AP) film does not. An AP **supine** film should arouse suspicion if there is lucency at the lung base with visualization of the anterior costophrenic sulcus (see Fig. 6-27).

6. When the distance from the inner rib to the medially displaced visceral pleura is 2.5 cm or greater, or the patient is exhibiting symptoms, needle aspiration in the anterior second intercostal space or chest tube insertion is indicated.

7. "Spontaneous pneumothorax" occurs in young, tall patients (late teens to thirties) or patients with COPD, and is caused by rupture of apical blebs; frequently this is a recurrent problem in these patients.

B. **Hemothorax**

1. Hemothorax cannot be distinguished radiographically from presence of other forms of pleural fluid (e.g., serous, chylous); when the trauma is significant, the fluid is assumed to be blood.

2. General guidelines for detection of small amounts of fluid

   a. Upright posteroanterior (PA) or AP blunting of lateral costophrenic sulci indicates 200 ml of pleural fluid.

   b. Upright lateral radiographic blunting of posterior costophrenic sulcus indicates 70 ml of fluid.

   c. Lateral decubitus view shows increase in pleural density—10 to 15 ml of fluid.

3. Traumatic hemothorax may result from lung injury or adjacent disruption of a nonpulmonary vessel; a **persistent hemothorax** is more likely caused by **nonpulmonary bleeding** (e.g., intercostal artery).

4. **Radiographic findings** (see Figs. 5-7, 5-31, and 7-2)

   a. **Supine films.** Generalized haziness of the affected hemithorax; the abnormal pleural fluid may collect superolaterally in the hemithorax.

   b. **Upright film.** Meniscus appearance or subpulmonic accumulation (latter mimics elevated hemidiaphragm).

## IV. Cardiac trauma

### A. Pericardial injury

1. Caused by either **blunt** (often steering wheel) or penetrating trauma.

2. **Cardiac tamponade** from hemopericardium is the **major complication.**

3. When venous return and diastolic filling are compromised and cardiac output decreases, emergency pericardiocentesis is warranted.

4. Fewer than 300 ml of rapid blood accumulation into the pericardium from the myocardial, pericardial, great vessel, or coronary arterial injury can result in cardiac tamponade.

5. **Plain film findings** (see Figs. 5-7 and 5-39)

   a. Frontal x-ray shows an enlarged globular cardiac silhouette.

   b. The **lateral chest x-ray** is positive in 50 percent of patients with significant pericardial effusion.

   c. The **major finding** on lateral chest x-ray is separation of epicardial fat from pericardial fat (greater than 2 mm) with abnormal water density representing the pericardial fluid.

   d. The frontal films may show this finding in about 25 percent of instances.

6. **Echocardiography** is an excellent method to detect pericardial effusion if the patient is stable.

7. Computed tomography (CT) also can detect pericardial effusion.

### B. Myocardial injury

1. Two major types of injury exist—**contusion and laceration.**

2. **Contusion** usually results from **steering wheel injury;** there is a high association with **fractures** of the **sternum** (Fig. 7-5).

3. Contusion may present in a fashion similar to myocardial infarction.

4. On chest x-ray, **cardiac aneurysm or pseudoaneurysm** may result from contusion.

5. **Penetrating myocardial injury**

   a. From stab or bullet wounds.

   b. Cardiac chambers and structures likely to be involved (in descending order of frequency): RV>LV>RA>LA> great vessels.

   c. **Pseudoaneurysm** may result if the patient survives.

   d. Acutely this injury may progress to cardiac tamponade, hemothorax, and shock.

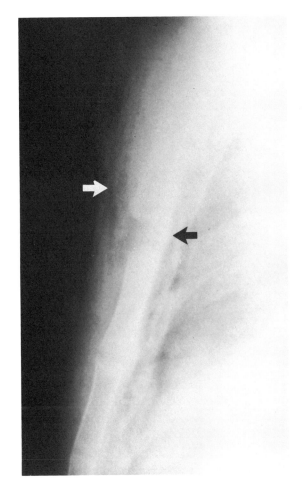

**Fig. 7-5.** *Fracture of the sternum portends more serious internal injury. The black arrow points to separation fracture of the manubrium and sternal body. Sternal fracture is associated with serious lung, heart, or vascular injury. The superficial linear lucencies (white arrow) indicate subcutaneous emphysema. This is due either to an open wound or dissecting injury to the trachea, bronchi, or lungs.*

    e. Bullets may lodge in the interventricular or interatrial septa, in cardiac walls, or in the atrial or ventricular chambers; in the latter case, they may embolize into the arterial tree.

**V. Thoracic aortic trauma**

  **A.** Injuries occur from **rapid deceleration,** chest compression, or falls from heights.

  **B.** Most common **sites of aortic tear** are the **aortic isthmus** (75% of instances), just distal to the takeoff of the left subclavian artery, and the **ascending aorta (20% of patients)**; the isthmus is nonmobile and subject to tearing and shearing forces.

  **C.** The intima and media usually are disrupted, while the adventitia often remains intact.

  **D.** Ascending aortic tears carry a worse prognosis than isthmus injuries. **All thoracic aortic injuries are serious,** however, **and are a major cause of instant death from motor vehicle accidents and from falls.**

**Fig. 7-6.** *In the setting of trauma, widening of the mediastinum (white arrow) suggests serious injury to the vessels or the thoracic spine from hemorrhage.* **A.** *In this patient, the aortic arch is partially obscured, heightening the suggestion of vascular injury.* **B.** *The aortogram demonstrates the intimal flap (black arrow) characteristic of an aortic tear.*

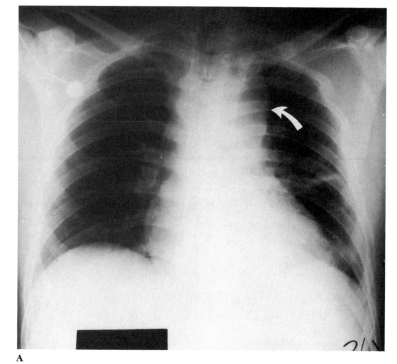

A

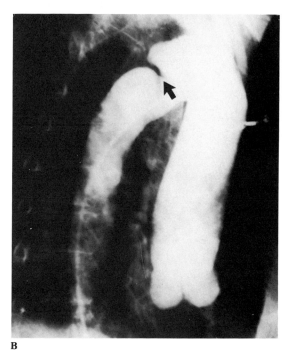

B

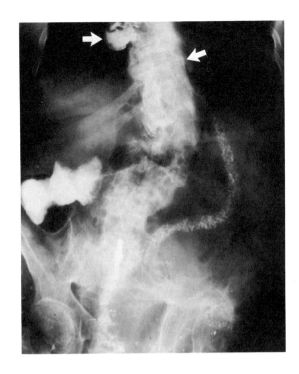

**Fig. 7-7.** *Diaphragmatic hernia may be acute or delayed following trauma. Barium enema in this patient demonstrated herniation of the colon into the thorax (arrows). This injury is more frequent on the left side.*

    E. **Chest x-ray findings** (Fig. 7-6)

        1. **Mediastinal widening.**

        2. **Obscuration** of the aortic contour, especially the **arch.**

        3. **Left apical "cap,"** caused by tracking of blood up and over the left lung and pleura.

        4. **Tracheal displacement** to the right.

        5. Associated **fractures** of the **upper** two ribs.

        6. A nasogastric tube becomes deviated to the right.

    F. CT with contrast enhancement has an increasing role in assessment of thoracic aortic injuries; angiography remains definitive, however.

  VI. **Diaphragmatic trauma**

    A. **Clinical aspects**

        1. Left hemidiaphragm affected more frequently than right.

        2. Caused by blunt or penetrating trauma to the chest or abdomen.

        3. Hernia may occur at time of injury or be delayed for months to years.

        4. Herniated contents may include stomach, large or small bowel, omentum, spleen, kidney, or liver.

    B. **Radiographic findings** (Fig. 7-7)

        1. Poor definition of hemidiaphragm.

        2. Abnormal air and fluid densities in the chest (bowel and stomach).

        3. May appear as elevated hemidiaphragm.

        4. Ipsilateral pulmonary atelectasis.

**5.** Barium studies help define whether enteric contents are in chest.

**VII. Skeletal trauma**

    **A.** Rib

        **1.** Rib fractures may be isolated and uncomplicated or may be multiple and associated with flail chest; they may portend other serious injuries.

        **2.** Specific rib fractures have different connotations

          **a. Rib fractures 1 to 3**

            **(1)** Associated with aortic tear or ruptured bronchus.

            **(2)** Associated mediastinal or pleural air suggests **ruptured bronchus.**

          **b. Rib fractures 4 to 9**

            **(1)** Frequently uncomfortable but not serious.

            **(2)** Hemopneumothorax is major complication, rather than injury to another organ.

            **(3)** If five or more ribs are fractured or if ribs are fractured in more than one site, flail chest may ensue.

          **c. Rib fractures 10 to 12**

            **(1)** Associated with abdominal injuries (especially liver, kidney, and spleen) (Fig. 7-8).

            **(2)** More **posterior** fractures increase likelihood of associated abdominal organ injury.

        **3.** Major direct **complications** of rib fractures

          **a.** Pneumothorax

          **b.** Hemothorax

        **4.** Costal cartilages, at the anterior ends of ribs, may be fractured and painful but are difficult to detect by radiography.

    **B.** Sternal fractures (Fig. 7-5)

        **1.** Best detected in the emergency room by lateral or oblique radiograph and tomograms (CT helpful when available)

        **2.** Associated with cardiac and pericardial injuries

        **3.** Occurs with blunt, compressive trauma (e.g., steering wheel)

    **C.** Scapular fractures (Fig. 7-9)

        **1.** Uncommon

        **2.** Associated with upper rib fractures

ABDOMINAL TRAUMA

**I. Splenic trauma.** When a patient presents in shock from traumatic splenic rupture, radiology plays no direct role. Short of the life-threatening situation, however, radiology frequently is crucial to the diagnosis of splenic injury as well as determination of its extent and associated injuries. In both blunt and penetrating trauma to the spleen, concomitant chest and liver injuries occur with increased frequency. Orthopedic,

**Fig. 7-8.** *Fractures of the posterior lower left ribs are associated with splenic and left kidney injuries. This patient sustained fractures of the ninth and tenth ribs (arrow) on the left. There was hemoperitoneum, and at surgery splenic rupture was found.*

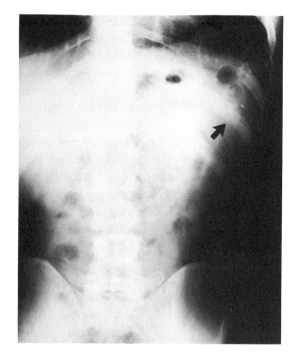

**Fig. 7-9.** *Scapular fracture. Note at least two fractures (arrows). This injury raises the suspicion of adjacent pulmonary and vascular injury.*

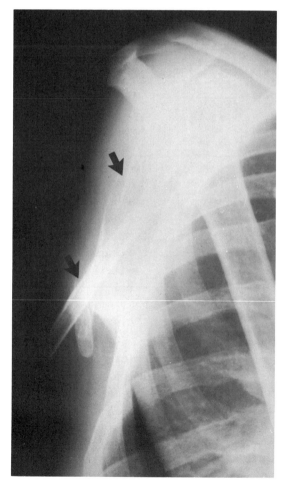

genitourinary, gastrointestinal, and craniospinal injuries also are associated, and the radiologic workup must be tailored accordingly.

Radiology findings in the acutely bleeding spleen may differ from those of the spleen with "delayed" rupture (i.e., a previously tamponaded injury "rebleeds"). Similarly, the various types of splenic injuries—frank rupture, subcapsular hematoma, contusion—often can be differentiated by radiographic criteria. This differentiation aids the now-important determination of which injured spleens may be observed and salvaged versus which require immediate operation. Pathologically enlarged spleens (e.g., from infectious mononucleosis, chronic myelogenous leukemia, malaria, polycythemia vera) are more susceptible to trauma.

A. **Plain film findings with ruptured spleen**
   1. **Caveats regarding plain films in ruptured spleens**
      a. **A normal plain film does not exclude major splenic injury.**
      b. **The most sensitive radiographic finding with splenic rupture—left paracolic gutter blood—is invalid if peritoneal lavage has been performed previously.**
   2. **Direct findings**
      a. **Separation of the lateral wall of the descending colon from the properitoneal fat stripe.** This indicates fluid **(blood)** in the **dependent left paracolic gutter** from the splenic injury. If the distance is greater than 3 mm with a moderately gas-filled colon, the sign usually is valid. (There are occasional false positives—see Chap. 6, Ascites.)
      b. **Extensive hemoperitoneum.** Signs similar to those of generalized ascites. This amount of blood usually signifies other major injuries as well (Fig. 6-47).
      c. **Enlarged splenic outline or left upper quadrant mass.** This indicates blood within the spleen itself or a subcapsular or perisplenic hematoma. A pathologically enlarged spleen without injury may have this appearance.
      d. **Ill-defined or hazy splenic margins.** In a patient with moderate body fat or in obese patients, the splenic outline should be sharp—lack of this outline may signify bleeding. **A prior abdominal film for comparison** may be helpful, as this finding may be subtle.
   3. **Associated findings**
      a. **Rib fractures.** Occur in approximately 15 to 20 percent of patients and less frequently in children. The

association is specifically with **left lower ribs 10 to 12,** usually in the posterior and axillary portions (see Fig. 7-8).

    **b.** Upper left vertebral **fractures** of the transverse processes.

    **c. Chest abnormalities.** These include left pneumothorax, hemothorax or hemopneumothorax, left lower lobe atelectasis or contusion, and elevation of the left hemidiaphragm.

    **d. Secondary findings involving the stomach**

        **(1)** Medial or inferior displacement of the stomach (or both)

        **(2)** Thickened gastric rugae in the fundus and along the greater curvature (dissection of blood and edema along the lienogastric ligament)

        **(3)** Gastric dilatation caused by ileus

    **e.** Depression of the splenic flexure of the colon.

    **f.** Findings suggesting left renal injury. There is a high incidence of associated splenic and left kidney trauma.

**B. Imaging and invasive studies in splenic trauma.** All patients with splenic trauma do not require confirmatory special studies such as ultrasound, CT, or angiography. In the appropriate clinical setting (without radiographs) or in the deteriorating patient with highly suggestive plain film findings, surgery should not be delayed. However, when the clinical, plain film, and peritoneal lavage findings are not diagnostic of splenic injury, these special radiographic studies usually will cinch the diagnosis. Similarly, when the patient is stable, these studies may delineate the degree and type of injury.

**II. The liver.** Most patients with major hepatic injuries bypass the radiology department, and rightfully so. The vulnerable hepatic veins and adjacent inferior vena cava make the liver subject to critical injury. As such, the tenet that shocky, potentially catastrophic patients should not be unattended in the radiology department is emphasized. Virtually all basic examinations can be performed portably in an area where resuscitative and stabilizing fluids and equipment are readily available.

For the patient who is not so critically injured, however, radiology can provide early and often pivotal information. Patients with hepatic injury may have few clinical signs or nonspecific right upper quadrant symptoms or may be comatose, obscuring the abdominal findings.

The liver that is enlarged, pathologically or physiologically (i.e., from tumor versus pregnancy), is more prone to injury. The right lobe of the liver is most commonly injured. High-velocity, high-volume gunshot wounds carry the highest mortality. Bursting injuries compared to simple lacerations carry a worse prognosis. "Spontaneous" nontraumatic rupture also occurs (e.g., in benign hepatic adenomas in female patients taking birth control pills).

Possible **findings on plain abdominal films include:**

A. **Direct hepatic findings**

    1. **Hemoperitoneum,** as in splenic injury, is the most sensitive indicator of intraperitoneal visceral rupture. Fluid in the right paracolic gutter is the earliest sign (Fig. 6-47). Unlike the spleen, which usually does not manifest massive free peritoneal fluid, liver injury can have frank signs of radiographic ascites (hemoperitoneum).

    2. **Enlarged liver.** This sign is valid only if the liver is unequivocally enlarged, with the lower margins below the iliac crest (not a Riedel's lobe configuration) and the left lobe extends across the midline. There is too much variation in normal livers to assign much significance to subtle enlargement. Previous comparison films that show a present increase in hepatic size are valuable (Figs. 6-16 and 6-17).

    3. **Abnormal hepatic contour.** Bulging of the liver margins, particularly a convex inferior margin, is often a more reliable sign of hepatic injury than size per se. Intrahepatic and subcapsular hematomas may cause focal bulges but leave the hepatic margin sharp.

    4. **Loss of sharp hepatic margins,** also seen with hemoperitoneum and frank capsular rupture.

    5. **Adjacent organ displacement** caused by intrahepatic, subcapsular, or perihepatic hematoma

        **a.** Stomach deviation to the left and anteriorly by the left lobe

        **b.** Hepatic flexure of the colon, inferiorly displaced by an enlarged liver or hematoma

        **c.** Diaphragmatic elevation caused by expanding liver

    6. Localized right upper quadrant or generalized **ileus.**

B. **Associated injuries** and signs in conjunction with liver trauma include:

    1. Right lower **rib fracture(s).** Usually posterior or in the axillary line

    2. **Chest**

        **a.** Elevated hemidiaphragm

        **b.** Hemopneumothorax

        **c.** Atelectasis or pulmonary contusion

        **d.** Ruptured hemidiaphragm with abdominal contents in the chest (may mimic simple eventration)

    3. **Loss of right psoas or renal contour** or both, with

right kidney fracture, or inferior displacement of the kidney by hepatic enlargement or hematoma.

C. **Special imaging studies in hepatic trauma.** The previously mentioned special imaging studies in suspected splenic trauma are pertinent for the liver as well. In addition, radionuclide liver-spleen scanning demonstrates both organs, and a combined liver-lung scan yields information about the right subphrenic space.

III. **The pancreas.** Pancreatic injuries occur less frequently than most other visceral injuries. Detection of pancreatic injury has been difficult because of the shielded, central position of the pancreas in the abdomen. Ultrasound and CT have assumed major roles in the morphologic depiction of the pancreas and its diseases.

Pancreatic and duodenal injuries frequently coexist because of the proximity of these organs. Blunt trauma from a steering wheel or bicycle handlebar or from contact sports accounts for most pancreatic injuries. Clinical diagnosis of pancreatic injury may be difficult; peritoneal lavage often is negative (because the pancreas is a retroperitoneal structure), and on occasion, serum amylase will be normal.

Although there are no specific plain film findings of pancreatic injury, constellations of abnormalities may be quite suggestive. The basic mechanism for most radiographic findings is pancreatic enzyme dissection with inflammation of adjacent mesenteries and ligaments. This causes localized ileus and mass effect from blood, edema, or pseudocyst.

Signs of fluid in the lesser sac often cannot be distinguished from signs of the abnormal pancreas itself. Patients may present at a time long after the initial injury with a traumatic pseudocyst if the pancreatic injury was not suspected initially.

A. Possible findings on abdominal films include:

1. **"Colon cutoff."** The transverse colon is variably distended to the region of the true splenic flexure of the colon (at the phrenicocolic ligament) because of transverse mesocolon and phrenicocolic irritation (Fig. 6-37).

2. **"Sentinel loop."** Localized duodenal or, less commonly, jejunal dilatation from inflammation of the mesenteric root (Fig. 6-37).

3. **Epigastric soft-tissue mass** from hematoma or edema (or, later in the course, pseudocyst) causing displacement of adjacent bowel or stomach.

   a. **Gastric displacement.** Usually anteriorly (a lateral film of the abdomen will better delineate anterior displacement); superior displacement of the stomach or soft-tissue impression on its inferior surface (Fig. 6-38).

      **b. Inferior displacement of the transverse colon** and increased distance between the stomach and transverse colon as the mass interposes itself.

      **c. Widening of the duodenal sweep** ("C-loop").

   **4.** The **psoas margins** may become **obliterated** because of adjacent retroperitoneal enzyme inflammation or bleeding.

   **5. Intraperitoneal hemorrhage** or pancreatic ascites or both will appear as ascites.

   **6.** Associated low anterior or posterior rib fractures as the result of blunt traumatic compression of the upper abdomen.

   **7.** Upper lumbar vertebral fractures.

 **B. Chest film** findings with pancreatic injury include:

   **1.** Pleural effusion (high amylase content), particularly left-sided.

   **2. Elevated left hemidiaphragm** and basilar subsegmental atelectasis.

   **3.** Lower **rib fractures** (chest and abdominal films should be meticulously checked).

   **4.** Pulmonary edema (rare).

 **C. Associated injuries** depend largely on the mode of injury and site of trauma. Injuries to the right of the vertebral column are more likely to involve the liver, duodenum, biliary structures, gastroduodenal artery, and, of course, the pancreatic head itself. Injuries to the left may involve the spleen and left kidney in addition to the pancreas. The kidneys usually need radiographic evaluation in pancreatic injury because of proximity.

 **D.** Notwithstanding the possible x-ray abnormalities previously mentioned, a normal film does **not** exclude pancreatic trauma. Conversely, in a patient being observed, **follow-up plain films** may show obvious changes and evolution. If pancreatic injury is strongly considered and plain films are inconclusive, further studies are warranted.

   **1. Gastrografin upper gastrointestinal series.** Water-soluble contrast will delineate the stomach and duodenal sweep, providing direct information regarding associated duodenal injury and indirect evidence of pancreatic injury (mass effect, edema, or blood) (Fig. 7-10).

   **2. Ultrasound and CT.** Both may depict the normal pancreas (and help exclude injury) or the abnormal pancreas (and prove injury). Ultrasound may be limited by bowel gas, and the tail of the pancreas frequently is difficult to visualize. Thus **CT is preferred.** Angiography is reserved for major vascular insult.

**IV. The genitourinary tract.** Renal trauma fortunately is not a

**Fig. 7-10.** *Duodenal–pancreatic head injury. The tapered narrowing of part of the duodenum (arrows) is characteristic of hematoma following trauma. This injury is not specifically seen on plain films, but requires an upper gastrointestinal series. Water-soluble contrast is used if perforation is suspected.*

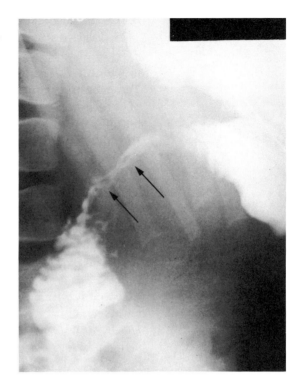

major cause of death. Frequently seen in conjunction with multiorgan injuries, most renal injuries are not severe. These include contusion and intrarenal or subcapsular hematoma. The surrounding renal capsule, perinephric fat (within Gerota's fascia), and retroperitoneum provide a tamponade effect, which helps stop bleeding.

Most renal injuries occur with blunt trauma, especially automobile and sporting accidents, and with altercations. Flank pain and hematuria are the cardinal findings; however, hematuria may be absent if the ureter is obstructed by clot. Kidneys with underlying abnormalities (e.g., congenital anomalies [pelvic kidney, crossed ectopia] or tumors) are more prone to injury. Injury to the renal vascular pedicle is serious and requires surgical correction. If the patient is stable, angiography provides a definitive diagnosis.

**Ureteral injuries** are most frequently iatrogenic (operative or occurring during cystoscopic maneuvers). **Bladder** and posterior urethral injuries commonly occur with blunt trauma and in association with pelvic fractures. Rapid deceleration with seat belts when the bladder is distended is a cause of bladder rupture. Instrumentation may cause vesicular injury as well. Bladder rupture may be intra- or extraperitoneal. Intravenous urography and cystography are the major modes for establishing diagnosis and determining the extent of these injuries.

CT provides valuable information and is assuming a greater role in diagnosis of genitourinary trauma. It differentiates intra- and extrarenal hematoma, demonstrates retroperitoneal blood, and shows injuries to pelvic structures that occur in association with bladder rupture. CT also provides simultaneous information about other abdominal organs that may be injured.

A. Findings that may be seen on plain films in renal trauma

1. **Loss or enlargement of the renal outline** caused by perirenal bleeding, intracapsular bleeding, or edema.

2. **Change in renal axis.** A localized hematoma may displace either the upper or lower pole away from the adjacent psoas muscle, which the kidney normally parallels.

3. **Soft-tissue mass** may be round or oval and is also the result of hematoma. Fluid-filled small bowel loops may mimic this appearance.

4. **Absence of psoas margin** caused by adjacent blood obliterating the fat planes. Because the psoas shadows may be absent normally, this is not a specific finding. An old film demonstrating the psoas margin makes absence on the present study more meaningful.

5. **Displacement of bowel** may occur as a result of hematoma.

6. Associated findings include **rib** or **transverse process fracture, scoliosis, paralytic ileus, and diaphragmatic elevation.**

B. **Indications for intravenous urography or pyelography (IVU or IVP) with suspected renal trauma**

1. Penetrating injury in the region of the kidneys.

2. Lower rib or transverse process fracture and microhematuria.

3. Hematuria.

4. Significant trauma without hematuria. A disrupted or clotted ureter may not permit hematuria to pass.

5. Preoperatively, awareness of anomalies that might be injured surgically (e.g., ureteral duplication) and of **presence and function of two kidneys** are important.

C. A 50-ml bolus of standard water-soluble contrast solution (e.g., Renografin 60%) will suffice for the intravenous urogram; to more accurately assess renal injury, however, nephrotomography is better. With minor injury such as contusion, the urogram most likely will be normal. Abnormal IVU findings that may be seen include:

1. **Lucent rounded or linear defect in the nephrogram,** caused by hematoma.

2. **Calyceal displacement** caused by the hematoma mass.

3. Poor **filling of the calyces** as a result of compression from edema or contusion.

**Fig. 7-11.** *Intravenous pyelographic findings in renal injury. Extravasation of contrast adjacent to the left kidney indicates visceral fracture involving the collecting system (arrow). The right side is normal.*

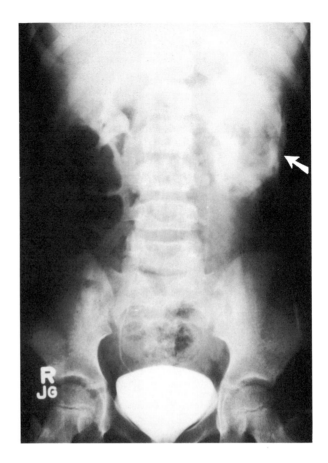

4. **Extravasation of contrast,** indicating a parenchymal tear involving the collecting system (Fig. 7-11).

5. **Poor or delayed visualization or nonvisualization** of the entire kidney is ominous and suggests vascular pedicle injury. It is an indication for angiography (depending on clinical status).

6. **Separate renal fragments or nonvisualization of part** of the kidney suggests a fractured or shattered kidney.

7. **Enlarged renal outline** in a functioning kidney results from obstruction of fluid flow from the kidney. This should arouse suspicion of an obstructed renal vein (thrombosis) or ureter (blood).

8. **Caveats**

   **a.** Shock will result in delayed visualization or nonvisualization of both kidneys.

   **b.** Kidney size and contrast excretion depend on baseline function of the kidneys, not just the acute event.

D. **Possible findings on IVU in ureteral injuries**

   1. Nonfunction or delayed function of the ipsilateral kidney

   2. Ureteral dilatation to the site of injury

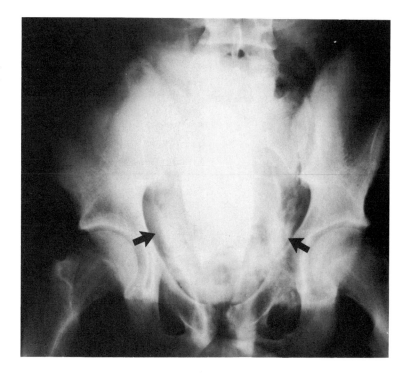

**Fig. 7-12.** *Bladder rupture. Cystogram demonstrates extravasation of contrast (arrows). The vertically elongated appearance of the bladder is caused by surrounding hematoma and urine. Fractures of the left ischial and pubic bones are seen and are frequently associated injuries.*

3. Extravasation

4. Ureteral deviation by an adjacent urinoma or hematoma

E. **Plain film findings with bladder and posterior urethral trauma**

1. Presence of a pelvic mass other than the bladder (perivesical fat distinguishes the bladder; see Fig. 6-18)

2. Gas in the bladder, especially with penetrating injury

3. Indistinct outline of the bladder

4. Adjacent pelvic fractures

F. **Findings on retrograde cystogram caused by bladder rupture**

1. **Intraperitoneal rupture.** Extravasated contrast flows into the cul-de-sac, around bowel loops, and may ascend into the lateral paracolic gutters.

2. **Extraperitoneal rupture.** Extravasated contrast remains perivesicular in the lower pelvis, generally in an irregular streaky configuration (Fig. 7-12).

3. Voiding urethrogram or retrograde urethrogram may be performed if urethral tear is suspected (see Fig. 3-7).

4. **Caveats**

a. Cystography should be performed under direct fluoroscopic vision and the procedure terminated when extravasation is seen.

b. Water-soluble contrast should be used.

c. Underfilling of the bladder with contrast (fewer than

200–300 ml) or lack of oblique films may yield false-negative results.

V. **Gastrointestinal tract.** Injuries to the gastrointestinal tract result in perforation or hematoma. Obstruction or ischemia may occur as a secondary problem. Penetrating injury commonly causes perforation, while blunt injury may cause hematoma or perforation or both. Seat belt injuries are associated with small bowel injury, particularly if the belt is strapped across the abdomen rather than the pelvis.

Anatomic relationships are important in understanding and predicting the results of injuries to the gastrointestinal tract. The second, third, and fourth portions of the duodenum, the ascending and descending portions of the colon, and the rectum are extraperitoneal. The remaining parts of the abdominal gastrointestinal tract (stomach, duodenal bulb, jejunum, ileum, transverse colon, colonic flexures, and part of the sigmoid colon) are **intra**peritoneal. Rupture of the latter structures causes acute peritonitis. Rupture of the gastrointestinal tract into extraperitoneal tissues results in more insidious abscess formation.

Radiographic findings of abnormal extraluminal gas or fluid (blood) in the peritoneum and retroperitoneum have been listed previously. More specific signs with trauma include:

A. **Possible findings with gastric injuries**
   1. **Perforation**
      a. Large amount of free air
      b. Ascites
   2. **Hematoma**
      a. Thick gastric rugae
      b. Gastric dilatation
      c. Displacement of the gastric air bubble
B. **Findings with duodenal injuries** (Figs. 7-10 and 7-13). Since the duodenum is largely retroperitoneal, duodenal injury generally does not result in free air. Duodenal and pancreatic injuries are commonly associated.
   1. Thickened duodenal (C-loop) folds
   2. Dilated proximal stomach and duodenum (to the site of hematoma)
   3. Abnormal extraluminal gas in the upper retroperitoneum
   4. Localized upper abdominal or diffuse ileus
   5. **Caveat.** Plain film findings are aided by water-soluble upper gastrointestinal series with suspected duodenal injury (especially perforation).
C. **Findings in jejunal and ileal injury**
   1. Free air does occur, but usually less than expected with gastric or colonic perforation.

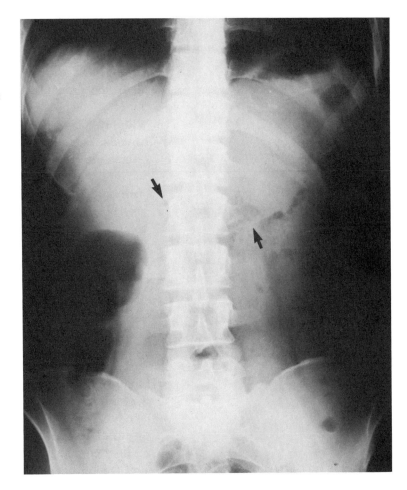

**Fig. 7-13.** *Pathological gas indicating post-traumatic duodenal injury. Abnormal streaks of retroperitoneal gas are the result of duodenal rupture (arrows). Most frequently the plain film is normal in appearance with duodenal rupture.*

    **2.** Thickened valvulae conniventes folds.

    **3.** Ileus or small bowel obstruction pattern.

**D. Findings with colonic injuries.** Findings depend on whether rupture occurs intra- or extraperitoneally. The cecum and sigmoid may rupture into either compartment.

    **1.** Large amounts of free or retroperitoneal gas

    **2.** Thickened, thumbprinted folds (better seen by barium enema)

    **3.** Bowel deviation by hematoma

    **4. Rectal injuries** cause

        **a.** Pelvic hematoma, which may deviate the bladder

        **b.** Streaky extraperitoneal pelvic gas

**VI. Intraperitoneal and retroperitoneal bleeding.** Intra- and retroperitoneal bleeding may be seen with injuries to any viscus or vessel. The findings of intraperitoneal bleeding mimic those of ascites.

    **A. Findings of intraperitoneal fluid**

        **1. "Dog-ears"**—rounded densities superolateral to the

bladder that represent dependent intraperitoneal fluid in the paravesicular fossae. This condition must be differentiated from fluid-filled bowel.

2. **Supravesical oval or rounded density** results from more fluid accumulating in the pelvis (cul-de-sac) and is not to be confused with the uterus.

3. **Widening of the density medial to the properitoneal fat stripe** (Fig. 6-47). This soft-tissue density represents intraperitoneal fluid between properitoneal fat and the lateral wall of the ascending or descending colon (anatomically, the paracolic gutters). Interposition of small bowel between the colon and flank stripe occurs in a small percentage of patients and can simulate this finding.

4. **Outward bulging and thinning of flank stripe** is caused by larger, clinically obvious, fluid distending the abdomen.

5. **Loss of spleen and liver margins.** Peritoneal fluid displaces these structures away from retroperitoneal and mesenteric fat; hence, margins of these organs are not seen.

6. **Floating of small bowel loops toward the center of the abdomen** is also a late finding with large amounts of fluid (Fig. 6-46).

7. **Generalized haziness.** This "ground-glass" appearance results from radiation scatter owing to the presence of large amounts of fluid.

B. **Findings with retroperitoneal fluid.** Retroperitoneal (extraperitoneal) fluid may accumulate in various potential spaces: **perirenal, anterior or posterior pararenal, paravertebral, or perivesical.** While the findings will vary with the location of the retroperitoneal fluid, the features common to all locations include:

1. **Loss of an expected outline.** The kidney or psoas muscle, for example, is seen because of the adjacent fat. If the fat is displaced or infiltrated by fluid or edema, the normal outlines will disappear.

2. **Displacement of a viscus** (the bladder by a hematoma, for example).

3. **Mass effect or density.** Seen in the area of the bleeding.

VII. **Gallbladder and biliary tree.** Gallbladder injuries are quite uncommon. In blunt trauma the gallbladder may become edematous from compromised blood supply rather than rupture. A right upper quadrant soft-tissue mass may be seen. Penetrating trauma can perforate the gallbladder of course, and intraperitoneal bile peritonitis may result. The common duct can become avulsed at the level of the pancreas with blunt trauma. Direct cholangiography or radionuclide imaging assesses its patency.

SELECTED READINGS

Cook DE, Walsh JW, Vick CW, Crewer WH. Upper abdominal trauma: Pitfalls in CT diagnosis. Radiology 159:65, 1986.

Danher J, Eyes BE, Kumar K. Oblique rib views after blunt chest trauma: An unnecessary routine? Radiology 156:262, 1985.

Federle MP. CT of upper abdominal trauma. Semin Roentgenol 19:296, 1984.

Goodman LR, Putman CE. S.I.C.U. chest radiograph after massive blunt trauma. Radiol Clin North Am 19:111, 1981.

Kaufman RA, Babcock DS. Approach to imaging the upper abdomen in the injured child. Semin Roentgenol 19:308, 1984.

Kuligowska E, Mueller PR, Simeone JF, et al. Ultrasound in upper abdominal trauma. Semin Roentgenol 19:281, 1984.

Marnocha KE, Maglinte DDT. Plain-film criteria for excluding aortic rupture in blunt chest trauma. AJR 144:19, 1985.

Marnocha KE, Maglinte DDT, Woods J, et al. Mediastinal-width/chestwidth ratio in blunt chest trauma: A reappraisal. AJR 142:275, 1984.

Marvis SE, Indeck M, Schorr RM, Diaconis JN. Posttraumatic tension pneumopericardium: "Small heart" sign. Radiology 158:663, 1986.

Mindelzun RE, McCort JJ. Upper abdominal trauma: Conventional radiology. Semin Roentgenol 19:259, 1984.

Reda EF, Lebowitz RL. Traumatic ureteropelvic disruption in the child. Pediatr Radiol 16:164, 1986.

Seltzer SE, D'Orsi CJ, Kirschner R, et al. Traumatic aortic rupture: Plain radiographic findings. AJR 137:1011, 1981.

# Pediatric Emergencies

*David C. Kushner*

Pediatric radiology in the emergency setting has important differences from standard adult radiology, including differences in technique, range, and variants of normal and disease entities. This chapter highlights the more common pediatric problems and the radiologic approach to their solution.

**I. Upper airway obstruction**

  **A. General considerations.** The severity of upper airway obstruction and stability of the pediatric patient determine the role of radiography.

    **1.** Inspiratory stridor, barking cough, ashen pallor, and hypoxemia indicate severe upper airway obstruction.

    **2. Direct clinical inspection** (with a tongue depressor) of the hypopharynx or epiglottis may cause agitation or **further obstruction** in the severely ill child. **Children with severe airway obstruction should not be radiographed.** Proper care necessitates transporting these children to an operating room where anesthesia, cautious endoscopy with endotracheal intubation, or controlled tracheostomy can be performed safely.

    **3.** Children with **mild or moderate** respiratory obstruction should be **accompanied** to the radiography suite by a **physician** equipped to deal with sudden airway emergencies. **No critically ill** (or imminently so) **child (or adult) should be left unattended in the radiology department.**

    **4.** The **principal causes** of pediatric upper airway obstruction include:

      **a. Epiglottitis** and supraglottitis

      **b. Foreign body**

      **c. Retropharyngeal abscess**

      **d. Viral croup**

  **B. Radiologic technical considerations**

    **1. Standard films** of the neck (assuming a stable patient) include:

      **a. Lateral view.** In slight extension and during late inspiration; may be performed with patient upright, supine, or in lateral decubitus position. This is the **most important view.**

    b. **Supine anteroposterior (AP) film.** Especially helpful for croup.

    c. Radiographs should stress soft tissues and hence be of lower kilovoltage.

2. **Normal variations** in the roentgenographic appearance of the airway may mimic severe obstructive abnormalities.

    a. **Flexion** of the neck on a lateral film **mimics retropharyngeal abscess** by causing the normal prevertebral soft tissues to appear thickened.

    b. **Lateral filming during expiration phase mimics retropharyngeal abscess.** The trachea bows anteriorly, and the retropharyngeal soft tissues thicken.

    c. **Swallowing** in the lateral view **mimics supraglottitis** by causing normal obliteration of air in the hypopharynx and larynx.

    d. **Expiration** phase in an AP film causes normal bowing of the trachea toward the side opposite the aortic arch (usually to the right), mimicking mediastinal or neck mass.

C. **Clinical entities and their radiologic diagnosis**

1. **Viral laryngotracheal bronchitis,** also called **viral croup**

    a. Approximate age range is 6 months to 5 years, with a peak at 2 years. (Croup may also occur in adults; the upper age range is not absolute).

    b. Usually preceded by an upper respiratory infection.

    c. Usually amenable to medical management. Occasionally severe obstruction requiring endotracheal intubation may occur.

    d. AP film is usually not necessary except to confirm the clinical diagnosis.

    e. **AP film** reveals **symmetric subglottic narrowing** from the lower surface of the true vocal cords to the **upper trachea** (Fig. 8-1). This narrowing does not change with phonation or respiration.

    f. **Lateral film** (Fig. 8-2) may reveal poor definition and slight narrowing of the subglottic air column. The lateral view is more useful for excluding other abnormalities than for diagnosing "croup."

2. **Supraglottitis** is also known in more limited form as "**epiglottitis.**" It is **most frequently caused by** *Hemophilus influenzae.* **Epiglottitis is an emergency situation.**

    a. Approximate age range is 2 to 8 years with a peak at approximately 5 years.

**Fig. 8-1.** *Viral croup on ontero-posterior (AP) film. Narrowing of the airway at the level of the sub-glottic larynx (arrows). Severe fixed tapering of the soft tissues with the apex at the true vocal cords.*

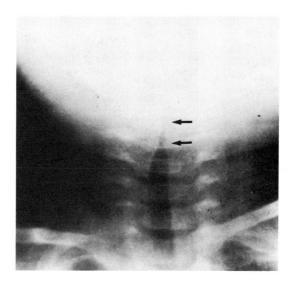

**Fig. 8-2.** *Viral croup on lateral film. Note normal hypopharynx, epiglottis (straight arrow), and retropharyngeal soft tissues, excluding epiglottitis and abscess. Hazy opacification of the sub-glottic air column with the loss of sharp definition of the margins of the trachea (curved arrow).*

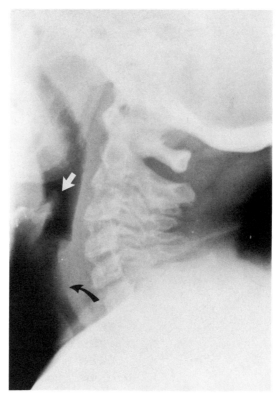

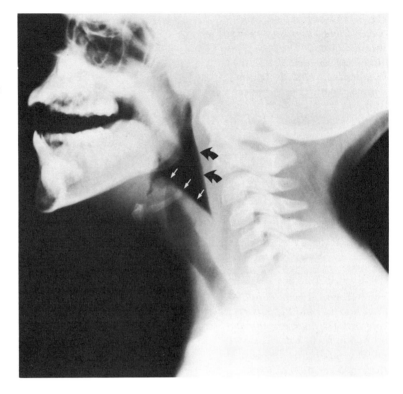

**Fig. 8-3.** *Supraglottitis including epiglottitis. Lateral film reveals dilation of the hypopharynx (curved arrows) and obliteration of the valleculae. Note marked swelling of the epiglottis and aryepiglottic folds (straight arrows) along with the false vocal cords.*

    **b.** Typically begins rapidly with progression to severe obstruction in a matter of hours.

    **c.** Usually produces severe air hunger, low-pitched stridor, high fever, polymorphonuclear leukocytosis, drooling, protruding mandible, and forward-leaning position.

    **d. Radiographic findings** on the **lateral film** include (Fig. 8-3):

        **(1) Dilatation** of the **hypopharynx**

        **(2) Swelling** of the **epiglottis** and **aryepiglottic folds**

        **(3) Edema** of the **vallecula** and **laryngeal ventricle**

        **(4)** Associated **subglottic swelling**

    **e. AP film** has no role when supraglottitis has been diagnosed in lateral view.

**3. Retropharyngeal abscess** may vary in presentation from mild "sore throat" to pain, high fever, and airway obstruction. Symptoms may mimic croup or bacterial epiglottitis.

    **a.** Children of any age may be affected, although most patients are between 2 and 10 years.

    **b.** Occasionally there will be a history of penetrating pharyngeal trauma. Most cases, however, occur from bacteremia (*Staphylococcus, H. influenzae, Streptococcus*).

**Fig. 8-4.** *Retropharyngeal abscess. Lateral film demonstrates marked thickening of the prevertebral soft tissues.*

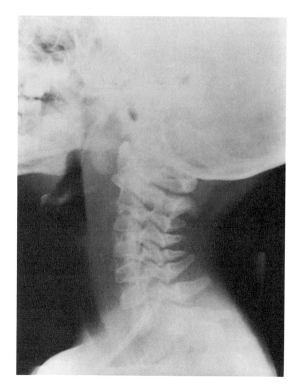

c. **Radiographic findings** on the **lateral film** include (Fig. 8-4):

    (1) **Straightening** or **reversal** of the **normal cervical lordosis** caused by prevertebral spasm and inflammation.

    (2) **Thickening** of the **retropharyngeal soft tissues** at the level of **C2** or **C3** (more than one-third to two-thirds of the sagittal diameter of a vertebral body).

    (3) Occasionally there will be **retropharyngeal gas.**

II. **Foreign body aspiration in the esophagus**

  A. **Clinical aspects** of foreign body aspiration or ingestion:

    1. Foreign body aspiration should be suspected in all children who can reach and grasp.

    2. Any unusual or prolonged respiratory symptoms should cause suspicion of foreign body aspiration.

    3. Children who ingest **esophageal** foreign bodies usually have **respiratory symptoms** similar to those that occur with aspirated airway foreign bodies (cough, stridor). Esophageal foreign bodies only rarely cause dysphagia or swallowing difficulty.

    4. A high index of suspicion is necessary because symptoms are quite variable and history may be poor.

  B. **Radiographic detection of the foreign body**

**Fig. 8-5A.** *Esophageal foreign body (coin). Lateral view shows coin overlying the cervical esophagus. One view does not prove its position in two dimensions.*
***B.** Esophageal foreign body (coin) on oblique view. The two films prove the esophageal location of the coin. The coin was present for 3 weeks and the only symptom was cough.*

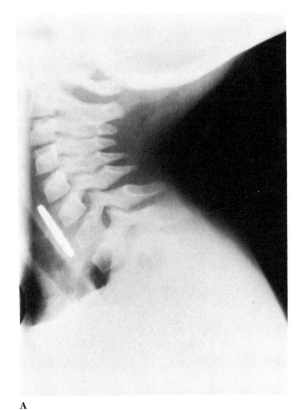

A

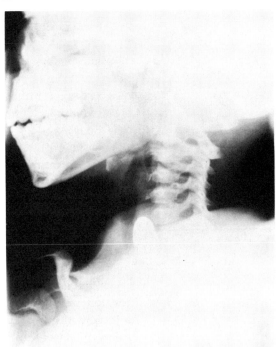

B

**Fig. 8-6.** *Aspirated endotracheal foreign body (peanut) in right bronchi. AP chest film demonstrates complete atelectasis of the right middle lobe (arrows). Note also obstructive emphysema of the right upper and lower lobes (hyperlucency in remainder of right lung) with the mediastinum shifted toward the left.*

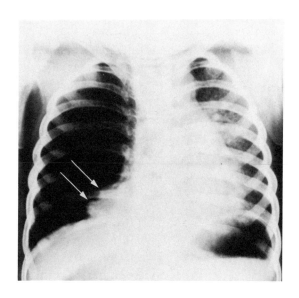

1. **Two projections** at right angles (AP, lateral, or oblique) are necessary for accurate **localization** of opaque foreign bodies (Fig. 8-5A and B).

2. **Radiolucent** foreign bodies can be recognized only by the **secondary abnormalities** that they may produce. Many children who have aspirated foreign bodies have normal radiographs and chest fluoroscopy; therefore, **normal examinations do not rule out foreign bodies** of the airway.

3. Esophageal radiolucent foreign bodies can be diagnosed only with contrast examination of the esophagus (usually barium).

4. Removal of esophageal foreign bodies with a balloon catheter under fluoroscopic guidance is a widely used technique.

C. **Secondary findings on chest x-ray from foreign body aspiration** (Fig. 8-6)

1. The foreign body may act as an endobronchial "ball valve" causing **overinflation** and **air trapping** in the segment or lobe involved.

2. The foreign body may totally **occlude** a bronchus, causing **atelectasis** of the corresponding lobe or segment.

3. Inspiration and expiration PA chest films or fluoroscopy may be necessary to detect subtle volume abnormalities.

   a. If there is **air trapping,** the **mediastinum** will shift **away** from the involved side at rest or during **expiration.** The foreign body prevents air from being expelled.

   b. If there is atelectasis without air trapping, the mediastinum will stay at midline or shift slightly toward the involved side on expiration.

4. Lateral decubitus chest films may be substituted for inspiration-expiration films if the patient cannot cooperate.

5. Chronic foreign body aspiration may cause chronic pneumonia, bronchiectasis, and failure to thrive.

### III. Specific pediatric chest problems

#### A. Bronchiolitis

1. Relatively common in children below 2 years of age.

2. Bronchiolitis is a **viral interstitial pneumonia** often caused by respiratory syncytial virus (RSV). It predominantly affects the peripheral bronchiolar airways.

3. **Clinically** there is tachypnea, hypoxemia, overinflation, and air trapping, which do not respond to bronchodilator therapy.

4. **Roentgenographic characteristics** are **unlike** those of most **other forms** of **pulmonary infection** (Fig. 8-7)

   a. Very large lung volumes; overinflation is documented repeatedly.

   b. Frequently, only slight thickening of the bronchial walls and radiating perihilar liner "streaking" is noted. Alternating areas of linear atelectasis and lobar or segmental overinflation (**irregular aeration**) may occur.

   c. **Consolidations** are notably **absent.**

   d. The **heart** may appear **small** because of dehydration or decreased venous return caused by the high intrathoracic pressure and volume.

   e. Both **pneumomediastinum and pneumothorax** are complications.

#### B. Round pneumonia

1. Pneumonia causing a "round" density on chest roentgenograph is relatively common in children over the age of 2 years.

2. The organism is usually *Pneumococcus,* although others have been implicated. This pattern is occasionally seen in chronic granulomatous disease of childhood or its variants.

3. In the early prodromal period before the classic fever, cough, and pain of pneumococcal pneumonia have appeared, the large spherical shadow may be misinterpreted as a mass or malignancy.

4. Radiograph will show a **smooth, spherical density** of variable size (from less than 1 cm to many centimeters) in any lobe of the lung. There is usually no associated adenopathy or pleural fluid (Fig. 8-8).

5. Rarely, a spherical pulmonary nodule will appear during **measles pneumonia** in a child who has previously re-

**Fig. 8-7.** *Bronchiolitis shown on AP (**A**) and lateral (**B**) films. Severe overinflation, flattened hemidiaphragms, and wide interspaces along with streaky perihilar bronchial thickening and irregular aeration are all characteristic of bronchiolitis. Lack of consolidation is also typical.*

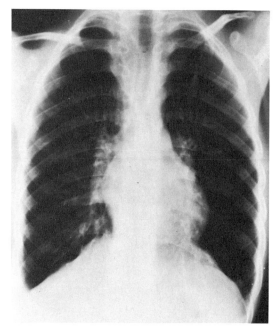

A

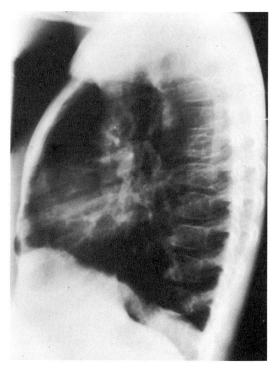

B

**Fig. 8-8.** *Round pneumonia on AP (**A**) and lateral (**B**) chest films in a 6-year-old child. Spherical masslike lesion in the right upper lobe. Sharp margins and hilar extension suggest neoplasm; however,* Pneumococcus *was cultured from the blood, and the film showed return to normal in 3 weeks.*

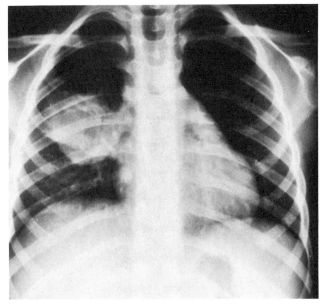

A

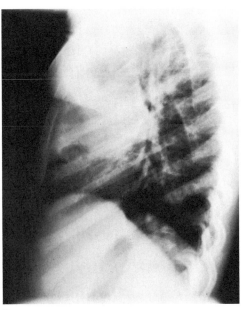

B

**Fig. 8-9.** *Diaphragmatic hernia. AP film reveals air-containing "cystic" structures in the left hemithorax. The left hemithorax is larger than the right, and there is shift of heart and mediastinum to the right. Note collapsed left lung pushed into the apex of the left hemithorax by the herniated bowel (arrows).*

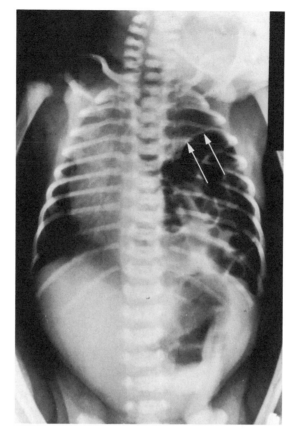

ceived attenuated measles vaccine. The round nodule will resolve spontaneously and should not be a cause for alarm.

6. If clinical symptoms compatible with bacterial pneumonia do **not** occur, other causes of pulmonary spherical densities should be considered (mass, granuloma, metastasis, sequestration).

C. **Diaphragmatic hernia**

1. **Congenital diaphragmatic hernia** occurs in utero and **presents as a surgical emergency** in the early **postnatal hours.**

   a. Congenital diaphragmatic hernia is more common than the noncongenital type.

   b. **Respiratory distress** and hypoxia are the predominant symptoms. Bowel sounds may be heard over the enlarged hemithorax.

2. The hernia occurs most frequently on the left side via the posterior foramen of Bochdalek.

3. Survival from diaphragmatic hernia is determined primarily by the maturity of the ipsilateral lung. The earlier in gestation (between 8 and 16 weeks) the hernia occurs,

the more immature and hypoplastic the lung will be at birth. If the hernia occurs later in gestation, the lung may be normal and survival ensured.

    **4. Roentgenographic abnormalities** include ( Fig. 8-9):

        **a.** Scaphoid, gasless abdomen

        **b.** Ipsilateral **dense hemithorax,** which may be entirely fluid-filled or a mixture of fluid and gas

        **c. Shift** of the **mediastinum away** from the hernia

    **5.** If the diagnosis is not apparent, it may be necessary to give barium or a small amount of air via a nasogastric tube to identify bowel loops in the chest. **Caution** must be taken since air or barium introduced into the bowel causes **expansion** of the loops in the chest and may further compromise the respiratory system.

  **D. Noncongenital diaphragmatic hernia** may occur following trauma, in children with neuromuscular disease or weakness, and, rarely, spontaneously in otherwise normal children.

    **1.** Physical signs and symptoms are similar to those of the congenital variety but much less severe.

    **2.** Diagnosis can be made by using the guidelines for congenital hernia.

**IV. Specific pediatric osseous problems**

  **A. Septic hip** is a **pediatric emergency** that may be associated with systemic sepsis and rapid destruction of the hip joint.

    **1.** Symptoms may be quite variable and **early clinical recognition difficult.** Septic hip may begin as **lethargy and fever,** with no localization of physical signs to the hip. Eventually, there will be **decreased range of motion, swelling,** and paradoxic irritability.

    **2.** Roentgenographic abnormalities may be quite subtle, and careful **technique** must be used.

        **a. Both hips** should be radiographed on the frontal film and the **gonads shielded.**

        **b.** Subluxation and effusion will be demonstrated best on **AP view. Frog lateral** view will best demonstrate position of the femoral head in reduction.

    **3. Radiographic signs** ( Fig. 8-10 )

        **a. Effusion and subluxation** are the **major findings.**

        **b.** An early but nonspecific abnormality may be lateral displacement of the fat planes adjacent to the hip.

        **c.** The **most reliable abnormality** is **subluxation of the femoral head laterally.** This is measured as the femoral head ( or neck )-to-teardrop ( acetabulum ) distance. This distance is usually symmetric ( less than

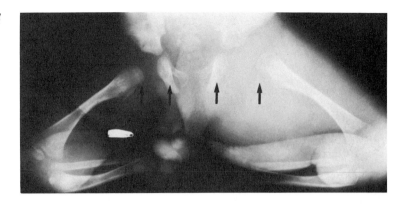

**Fig. 8-10.** *Septic hip. Frog lateral view of hips. The right hip is normal. Left hip and thigh soft tissues are markedly dense from inflammation. The left femur is dislocated laterally and superiorly. The left femoral neck-to-teardrop (medial acetabulum) distance is grossly asymmetric (arrows) compared to the right.*

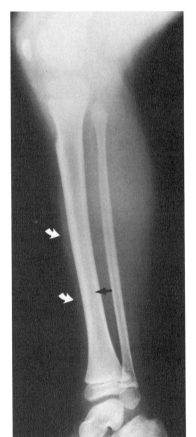

**Fig. 8-11.** *Toddler's fracture on lateral tibial film. Subtle but definite edema, irregularity, and blurring of the pretibial soft-tissue fat-muscle planes (curved arrows), compared to sharp posterior calf soft tissues. Vague suggestion of linear fracture line in distal tibia (straight arrow). The fracture may not be seen on the initial examination.*

2 mm difference between the hips) and is relatively independent of minor degrees of rotation.

    d. Actual **dislocation** of the hip **may occur;** it is usually lateral, superior, and dorsal.

    e. An ominous finding is **decreased joint width.** This late finding implies invasion and destruction of femur and acetabulum with hematogenous spread.

**B. Toddler's fracture**

  1. This is a **stress fracture** of the **midtibial shaft.** It occurs when a child begins to walk (toddle).

  2. Symptoms may consist of **irritability** and **refusal to use the extremity.**

  3. Physical findings are often nonspecific and difficult to elicit, and the diagnosis requires a high index of suspicion.

  4. The **diagnosis** can be correctly made by physical examination (if the child can be distracted); there is point tenderness over the midtibial shaft.

  5. **Roentgenographic abnormalities** may be quite subtle (Fig. 8-11)

    a. The initial finding of a nondisplaced fracture is **pretibial edema** of the soft tissues, seen on the **lateral** projection. Frequently the fracture lucency will not be visible for several days.

    b. When visible, a spiral fracture lucency without displacement may be seen in the midtibial shaft.

    c. Occasionally, films taken 10 to 14 days after the incident will reveal periosteal reaction, sclerosis, and healing when no fracture was suspected originally.

**C. Child abuse**

  1. Child abuse is unfortunately frequent but difficult to diagnose unless one has a **high index of suspicion.**

  2. Over half of abused children have no roentgenographic skeletal or soft-tissue abnormalities.

  3. Child abuse should be suspected when there are **unusual injuries** (e.g., pancreatic pseudocyst, focal burns).

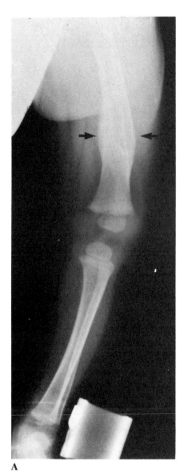

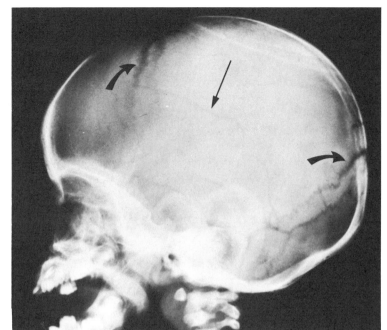

B

A

**Fig. 8-12.** *A. Examples of child abuse in different patients. AP film of left upper leg shows mid-femoral shaft fracture (arrows) at least 3 weeks old. Film was obtained because of cutaneous burns. B. Lateral skull films reveal linear frontotemporoparietal skull fracture (straight arrow). Note also widened cranial sutures (curved arrows) indicating increased intracranial pressure and volume from acute subdural hematoma. Parents admitted to previous episodes of child abuse.*

4. Skeletal radiographic findings suggestive of child abuse include ( Fig. 8-12A and B ):

   **a. Fractures of different ages.** Recognized as fractures without callus (healing) or fractures with mature callus (healed)

   **b. Fractures of unusual sites.** Vertebral body compression fractures, ribs (particularly the anterior ends), or both knees

   **c.** Fractures that may have occurred during **rotatory or shaking injuries.** Salter type I or II of femoral, tibial, or humeral growth plates ( Table 8-1 )

5. Child abuse may also be manifested by soft tissue injury of the brain (subdural hematoma, contusion) or by abdominal injuries to the liver (hematoma), spleen (rupture), kidney (laceration), or pancreas (hemorrhage or pseudocyst).

**D. Lead poisoning**

1. Remains epidemic in many areas of the United States.

2. **Acute lead intoxication** should be suspected in a child who presents with **vomiting, lethargy, encephalopathy, and coma.**

3. **Chronic** lead intoxication ( more than 6 weeks ) causes **mild retardation** or **failure to thrive, with anemia.**

**Table 8-1.** *Salter-Harris Classification of Fractures Involving the Epiphysis*

| Classification | Radiographic findings |
| --- | --- |
| Salter I | Soft tissue swelling and widening of epiphyseal plate or dislocation of epiphysis relative to metaphysis; films may appear to be normal except for soft tissue swelling |
| Salter II | Fracture apparent, extending into metaphysis |
| Salter III | Fracture apparent, extending across the epiphysis |
| Salter IV | Fracture apparent, extending across the epiphysis and into the metaphysis |
| Salter V | Soft tissue swelling only; compression of epiphyseal plate not seen radiographically |

    4. **Acute lead intoxication** has two **roentgenographic characteristics:**

        a. The **abdominal film** may reveal actual **lead particles** or metal flakes **within the bowel lumen** (Fig. 8-13A).

        b. **Skull examination** may reveal **widening** of the **cranial sutures** from cerebral edema and increased pressure (Fig. 8-13B).

    5. **Radiographic findings in chronic lead intoxication** (Fig. 8-14)

        a. Characteristic **dense bands of ossification** that incorporate the **zone of provisional calcification of the growing metaphysis.**

        b. Dense bands are seen in **all growing bones,** especially knees, wrist, proximal humerus, rib ends, and iliac crests.

**V. Specific pediatric abdominal problems**

  **A. Intussusception**

    1. **"Idiopathic" intussusception** is most common between the ages of **6 months and 2 years.**

    2. **Neonates** (less than 6 months old) and children **older than 3 years** have intussusception infrequently. In these age groups, many instances are caused by masses (polyps, lymphoma, duplication) acting as **"lead points."**

    3. **Symptoms** of intussusception usually occur in an otherwise well child. There is sudden spasmodic pain, drawing up of the legs, and vomiting. Initially normal stools are followed by passage of either **fresh or clotted blood (currant-jelly stool).**

    4. **Physical examination** usually reveals a **tender sausage-shaped mass** in the abdomen—usually **right lower quadrant.** If the signs of peritonitis or bowel ischemia are present, surgery should be performed immediately.

**Fig. 8-13. A.** *Examples of acute lead poisoning. Note several tiny flecks of radiopaque material (arrows) in the ascending colon on supine abdominal film. These are lead paint flakes in a child who was comatose from lead encephalopathy.* **B.** *Lateral skull film demonstrates abnormally large head size in this patient. The sutures are markedly widened (arrows) because of pressure from acute lead encephalopathy.*

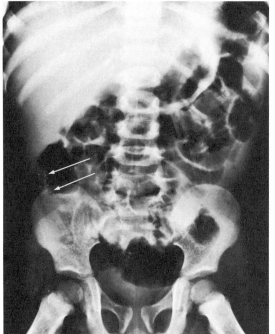

A

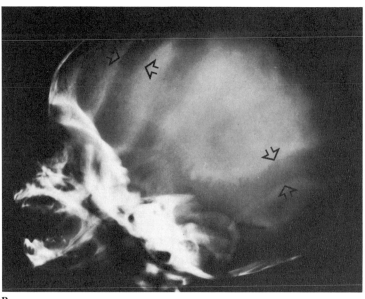

B

276

**Fig. 8-14.** *Chronic lead poisoning. AP film of the growing knee demonstrated dense bands. Dense bands in tibia and femur may be seen in normally stressed children; however, the fibular metaphyseal band is virtually diagnostic of heavy metal intoxication (arrows).*

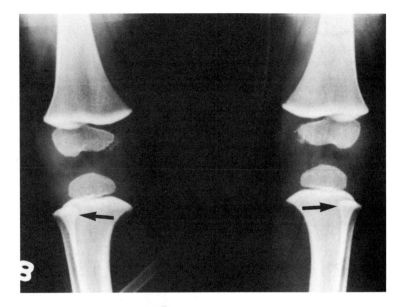

5. The radiographic contribution to intussusception may be both diagnostic (plain film and barium enema) and therapeutic (barium enema) (Fig. 8-15A and B):

a. Abdominal radiograph may be **normal.**

b. Abdominal findings include:

(1) **Right lower quadrant mass**

(2) **Small bowel obstruction**

(3) "Cutoff" (absence) of colonic gas in the midtransverse colon suggesting proximal colonic obstruction

6. If the child is clinically stable, has no sign of peritonitis or infarction, and has not been intussuscepted for a prolonged period of time, **diagnostic barium enema** should be performed by an experienced radiologist. If present, intussusception is documented by

a. Obstruction to retrograde flow of barium at the lead point (usually transverse or ascending colon)

b. "Coiled spring" appearance of barium flowing between the wall of the colon and folds of the mass that has intussuscepted

7. If an experienced radiologist who is trained in the technique of reduction is available, hydrostatic reduction of the intussusception may be attempted. Success is most frequent in the age group with idiopathic intussusception. Inexperienced personnel should not attempt intussusception reduction.

B. **Malrotation with volvulus**

1. Intestinal malrotation includes a complex group of em-

**Fig. 8-15.** *A. Intussusception. Plain film demonstrates multiple dilated loops of small bowel progressing toward the right lower quadrant, which is relatively gasless. This picture is diagnostic of small bowel obstruction.* **B.** *Intussusception diagnosed on barium enema. Note obstruction of retrograde flow of barium at the midtransverse colon. The barium column demonstrates the filling defect of the intussuscepted ileum (arrows) and the coiled-spring appearance of the barium at the interface.*

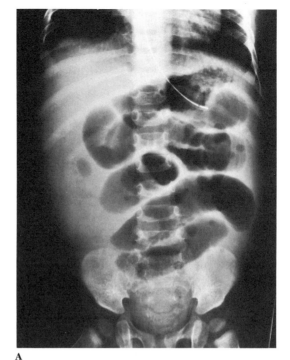

A

B

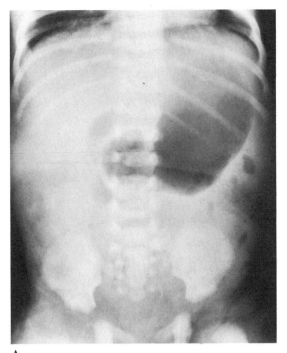

A

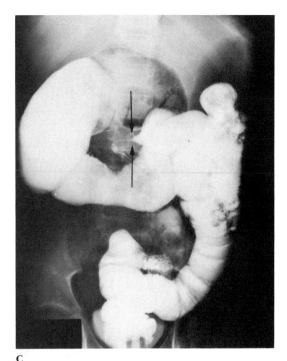

C

**Fig. 8-16. A.** *Malrotation with volvulus. Preliminary film reveals gas in stomach and proximal duodenum with relatively little gas distal to the third portion of the duodenum.* **B.** *Limited barium study demonstrates the point of volvulus and obstruction at the duodenal level of the superior mesenteric artery (straight arrow). Note the faint trickle of barium into small bowel in the* **right** *(rather than left) upper quadrant of the abdomen (curved arrow).* **C.** *Malrotation with volvulus. Barium enema in a different patient demonstrates flow of barium through descending and transverse colon with the hepatic flexure looped back on itself (malrotated). The actual point of volvulus is in the ascending colon, projected over the midlumbar spine (arrows). The cecum was located in the* **left** *lower quadrant.*

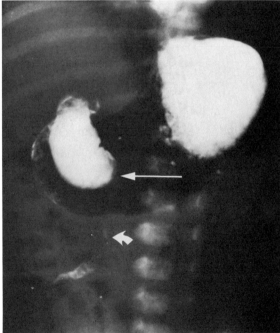

B

bryonic abnormalities. There is **abnormal position** of small and large bowel and **abnormal mesenteric fixation** of the bowel to the posterior abdominal wall.

2. **Abnormal** deficient mesenteric **fixation** is the cause of volvulus of colon or small bowel. **Volvulus complicating malrotation** may become an **emergency.** In the absence of volvulus, malrotation is an anatomic curiosity that may be treated electively.

3. Symptoms and signs of volvulus include **bilious vomiting, dehydration, and abdominal pain and tenderness.** If undiagnosed, the child will develop subsequent ischemia, infarction, and peritonitis.

4. Radiographic abnormalities may include:
   a. Small **bowel obstruction**
   b. Layering of dilated loops and air-fluid levels

5. **Upper gastrointestinal barium** examination via a nasogastric tube is the initial **method of choice** ( Fig. 8-16A and B ).
   a. Obstruction to barium flow at the second or third portion of the duodenum
   b. "Corkscrew" appearance of the duodenum as it demonstrates the volvulus around the mesenteric vessels
   c. Absence of the ligament of Treitz and location of the duodenum and jejunum in the **right** upper quadrant of the abdomen

6. **Barium enema** examination may also achieve diagnosis if the cecum and right colon are found to be in the **left** lower quadrant of the abdomen of if there is volvulus with obstruction and "beaking" of the midtransverse colon (as in total midgut volvulus) ( Fig. 8-16C ).

SELECTED READINGS

Eklof OA, Hartelius H. Reliability of the abdominal plain film diagnosis in pediatric patients with suspected intussusception. Pediatr Radiol 9:199, 1980.

Ellerstein NS, Norris KJ. Value of radiologic skeletal survey in assessment of abused children. Radiology 157:282, 1985.

Farnsworth PB, Steiner E, Klein RM, et al. Value of routine preoperative chest roentgenograms in infants and children. JAMA 244:582, 1980.

Gaisie G, Dominguez R, Young LW. Comparison of AP supine vs PA upright methods of chest roentgenography in infants and young children. J Nat Med Assoc 76:171, 1984.

Haller JO, Solvis TL. *Introduction to Radiology in Clinical Pediatrics.* Chicago: Year book, 1984. P. 206.

Kaufman RA, Towbin RB, Babcock DS, et al. Upper abdominal trauma in children: Imaging evaluation. AJR 142:449, 1984.

Oestreich AE. *Pediatric Radiology: Medical Outline Series.* New York: Medical Examination Publishing Company, 1980. P. 404.

Radkowski MA, Merten DF, Leonidas JC. Abused child: Criteria for the radiologic diagnosis. RadioGraphics 3:262, 1983.

Schultz RD, Willi U. Sonography after blunt abdominal trauma in childhood. Radiology 152:255, 1984.

Swischuk LE. Anterior displacement of $C_2$ in children: Physiologic or pathologic? Helpful differentiating line. Radiology 122:759, 1977.

# 9  Radiologic Special Procedures

*Eric vanSonnenberg*

The emergency physician should be aware of the array of special radiologic procedures and techniques and how to maximize and apply their information. These examinations are the diagnostic procedure of choice in many cases. Some of these studies are performed by specialized radiologic technologists. Interpretation of the studies requires a radiologist, and many of the procedures are performed by radiologists.

In the first part of the chapter, indications for the examinations will be emphasized, as this is most valuable for the emergency physician. The choice of these studies depends on availability and expertise at individual hospitals. The second part outlines new therapeutic options for acute disorders offered by interventional radiology techniques.

I. **Specific techniques and applications**
    A. **Nuclear medicine.** Nuclear medicine is useful as a diagnostic screening tool. The injection of specific radionuclide tracers that localize and are detected in specific organs or structures forms the basis of these studies. Radiologists or other trained physicians are needed to interpret the studies. Technologists handle the agents and inject the material. The appropriate emergency room uses of nuclear medicine examinations include:
        1. **Liver-spleen scanning.** In suspected intraparenchymal, subcapsular, or frank rupture of either of these organs, scanning is a relatively rapid and fairly reliable method of diagnosis (Fig. 9-1). Interpretation can be subtle, as false positives and negatives may occur, in part due to anatomic variations. The trained eye will minimize diagnostic errors.
        2. **Lung scanning for suspected pulmonary embolism.** The obstruction to radioactively tagged particles by embolic fragments in tiny pulmonary vessels results in an abnormal lung scan. Other nonembolic pulmonary diseases also may cause an abnormal scan; thus ventilation scans supplement perfusion studies for improved accuracy ( Fig.

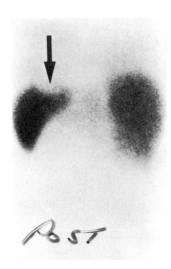

**Fig. 9-1.** *Perisplenic hematoma on posterior radionuclide scan. Technesium sulfur colloid liver-spleen scan demonstrates defect (arrow) along the superior margin of the spleen.*

9-2). An unequivocally negative scan reliably excludes pulmonary embolism.

3. **Biliary scanning.** New agents that are secreted normally by the liver and pass into the gallbladder and down the bile duct are helpful to diagnose cystic or bile duct obstruction.

4. **Testicular scanning.** Radionuclide scanning may be helpful to differentiate acute testicular torsion from acute epididymitis.

5. **Gastrointestinal bleeding.** Tagged red blood cells are used to diagnose blood pooling in the gastrointestinal tract caused by bleeding (Fig. 9-3).

6. **Meckel's diverticulum scanning.** This is a specific application of scanning for gastrointestinal bleeding. If the diverticulum contains gastric mucosa and is bleeding, the bleeding may be detected.

B. **Ultrasound.** This noninvasive technique has many emergency room applications, particularly in the abdomen and pelvis. A major benefit of ultrasound (US) is the lack of ionizing radiation, allowing its use in pregnant women and in children. A radiologist or technologist is required to perform the study; interpretation is done by a trained radiologist. US is limited by overlying bandages, bones, or abdominal gas.

1. Diagnosis of suspected **abdominal aortic aneurysm.** The outer diameter and often the size of the inner lumen of the aorta can be determined (Fig. 9-4). Involvement of the renal and other visceral arteries requires angiographic assessment. Iliac artery aneurysm also may be screened by US.

2. **Pelvic pain** in a woman of childbearing age. Ectopic pregnancy (Fig. 9-5), ruptured or nonruptured ovarian cysts, pelvic inflammatory disease, dermoid tumor, and endometriosis all may be detected as a mass lesion. Specific diagnosis often is not possible and must be correlated with clinical information. Intrauterine pregnancy (Fig. 9-6) and complications such as abruption and blighted ovum (Fig. 9-7) may be diagnosed.

3. **Hydronephrosis.** Obstructive uropathy is readily diagnosed by detection of dilatation of the renal collecting system; the degree of dilatation can be determined as well (Fig. 9-8).

4. **Biliary obstruction.** US is quite sensitive to both intra- and extrahepatic biliary obstruction (Fig. 9-9) and is excellent for its diagnosis or exclusion. The level and etiology of obstruction occasionally are determined; however, direct cholangiography and/or computed tomography often are required for further detail.

**Fig. 9-2.** *Radionuclide perfusion lung scan demonstrates decreased perfusion at the lung bases due to pulmonary emboli (arrows).*

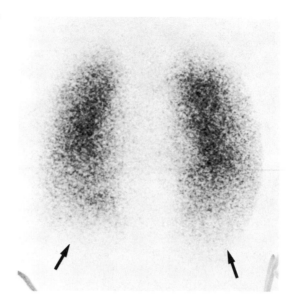

**Fig. 9-3.** *Focal accumulation of radionuclide in the right lower quadrant denotes a bleeding site in the ileum (arrow).*

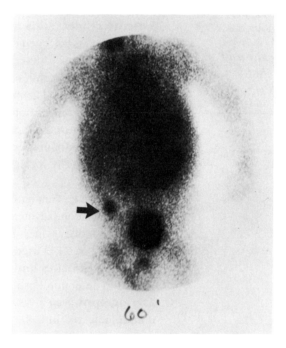

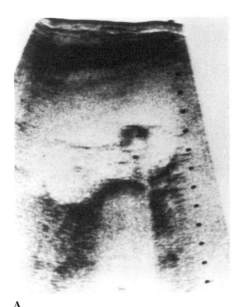

A

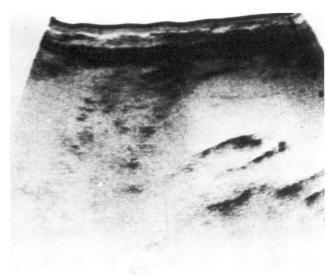

B

**Fig. 9-4.** *Sonographic demonstration of large abdominal aortic aneurysm that had dissected previously. Both the outer wall of the aneurysm and the inner true lumen are visualized on these transverse (A) and parasagittal (B) scans.*

5. **Acute cholecystitis and cholelithiasis.** The detection of gallstones has been revolutionized by US. A dilated gallbladder is easily determined by US as well. Other nonspecific, but helpful signs (such as pericholecystic fluid and a thick-walled gallbladder) occasionally may aid in the diagnosis of acute cholecystitis.

6. **Intraabdominal abscess.** Sonographic scanning and detection of abdominal compartments and viscera where abscesses typically localize is a well-established value of US (Fig. 9-10).

7. **Hematoma.** Traumatic or nontraumatic hematoma in peritoneal compartments or in parenchymal organs (liver, spleen, kidney) may be detected by US. Radionuclide scanning or CT is used more frequently for this purpose.

8. **Pleural effusion and ascites.** US is extremely sensitive for the detection of small amounts of fluid.

C. **Angiography** is an invasive procedure in which contrast medium is injected into the arterial or venous system through catheters placed percutaneously by a radiologist. In trauma, angiography frequently is the definitive diagnostic examination. Its use must be tailored to the clinical stability of the patient. Shocky patients are taken directly to the operating room. The increasing role of CT in trauma has reduced the use of angiography. The major indications for angiography in the emergency setting include:

1. Suspected traumatic **vascular injury,** either for diagnosis or to determine extent of the injury (especially thoracic aorta or arterial laceration of an extremity).

**Fig. 9-5.** *Ruptured ectopic pregnancy. Transverse sonogram demonstrates irregular hypoechoic blood in the cul-de-sac and in both adnexal regions (arrows). Typically, the ectopic gestation is not seen, which is the case in this patient. (U = uterus)*

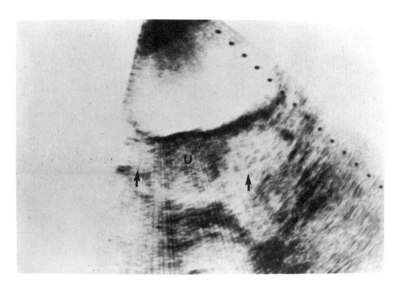

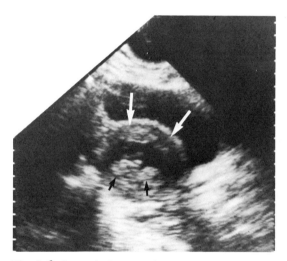

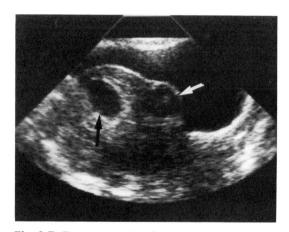

**Fig. 9-6.** *An early intrauterine pregnancy is visualized on this sonogram. The head and body of the fetus (black arrows) are identified within the gestational sac (white arrows).*

**Fig. 9-7.** *Empty gestational sac and fibroid. There is an abnormal irregular gestational sac without any identifiable fetal parts in this woman with first trimester bleeding (black arrow). A fibroid projects from the uterus and pushes into the bladder (white arrow).*

**Fig. 9-8.** *Sonographic demonstration of moderate dilatation of the calices, infundibulae, and renal pelvis in a patient with a stone obstructing the distal ureter. The kidney is outlined (arrows).*

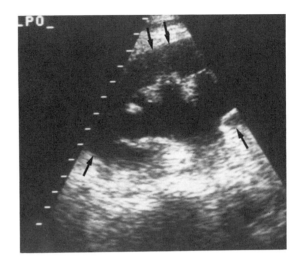

**Fig. 9-9.** *Dilatation of the common hepatic duct is demonstrated on this parasagittal right upper quadrant sonogram. Landmarks to identify the bile duct (open arrows) are the hepatic artery (arrowhead) and the more posterior portal vein (arrows).*

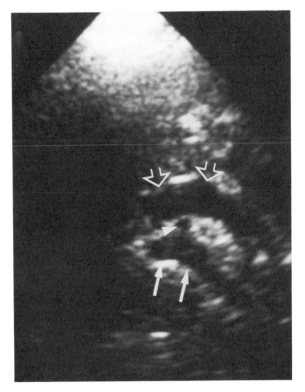

**Fig. 9-10.** *Transverse ultrasound examination displays two large intrahepatic abscesses (arrows).*

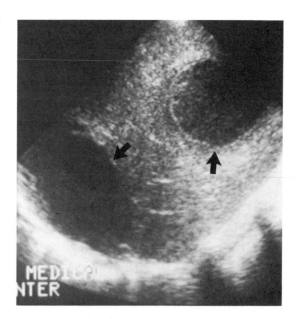

**Fig. 9-11.** *A large aneurysm of the hepatic artery is diagnosed by this arteriogram.*

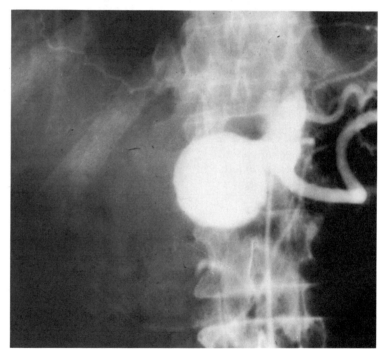

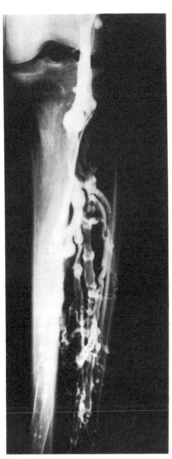

**Fig. 9-12.** *Multiple clots are noted as filling defects on this venogram of the lower leg.*

2. Suspected intraabdominal **visceral trauma,** especially splenic, hepatic, or renal injuries. Angiography is becoming an alternative, as CT is assuming a primary role.

3. Aortography in suspected nontraumatic thoracic or abdominal aneurysm ( Fig. 9-11 ) and **aortic dissection.** The examination is diagnostic for dissection, determines true and false lumen size, and assesses involvement of branch arteries.

4. Venography of the legs for suspected phlebothrombosis and **thrombophlebitis** ( Fig. 9-12 ).

5. Pulmonary angiography for suspected **pulmonary embolism** ( Fig. 9-13 ). Nuclear techniques are utilized initially for screening; angiography is definitive and reserved for equivocal data. Negative nuclear medicine screening studies are considered reliable.

6. In **gastrointestinal bleeding,** angiography may pinpoint the bleeding vessel ( Fig. 9-14 ). Intraabdominal drug infusion or embolization of particles may be used therapeutically to halt the bleeding.

D. **Computed tomography** (CT) has had extensive impact in diagnosis in current medical practice. It is a process by which serial tomographic slices (usually transverse) are displayed. These are reconstructed by a computer from data obtained by rotating x-ray tubes and multiple detectors. CT is considered invasive when IV contrast is utilized (as it is in most studies for trauma). Two general types of CT exist, based on body site: computed cranial tomography and computed body tomography.

**CT has become the major diagnostic procedure in head trauma.** It resolves the clinical dilemma of the importance of the presence or absence of a skull fracture, since the cranial contents themselves are depicted. **CT is indicated for suspected subdural** ( Fig. 9-15 ), **epidural** ( Fig. 9-16 ), **or intracranial hematoma,** as well as with depressed skull fractures. The study should be carried out as soon as possible after the injury for expeditious institution of proper therapy.

Injury to parenchymal organs (spleen [Fig. 9-17], liver, kidney [Fig. 9-18]) is well depicted by CT. Intra- and retroperitoneal blood and air, thoracic and abdominal aortic dissection, thoracic trauma, and injuries to vertebrae and the pelvic bones are well seen by CT.

CT yields important information if peritoneal lavage is positive, since it will demonstrate the actual site and extent of injury in most cases. Conversely, peritoneal lavage may be negative, yet a major retroperitoneal or intraparenchymal injury may be present ( Fig. 9-19 ); CT is extremely important

**Fig. 9-13.** *Large clots are seen in the left main pulmonary artery and its early branches in a patient with massive pulmonary embolism (arrows).*

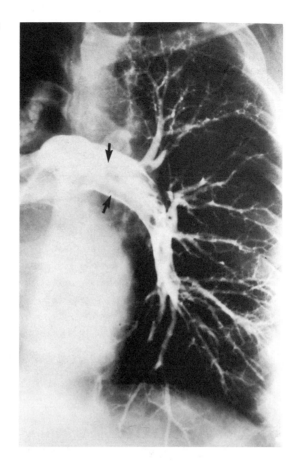

**Fig. 9-14.** *Inferior mesenteric arteriogram demonstrates distal bleeding vessel (arrow). The bleeding was halted by arteriographic embolization.*

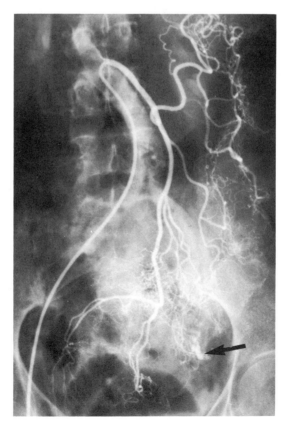

**Fig. 9-15.** *A large acute and chronic subdural hematoma is seen on this CT scan. There is compression of the ventricles and shift of the midline structures.*

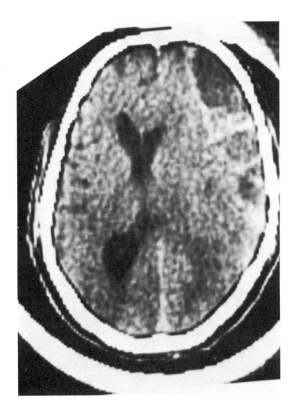

**Fig. 9-16.** *The bright density represents an acute epidural hematoma. There is mass effect with shift of the ipsilateral ventricle across the midline.*

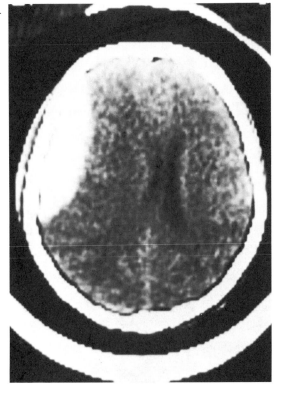

**Fig. 9-17.** *The low density defect within the spleen represents a large intrasplenic hematoma in this patient who suffered major trauma (arrows).*

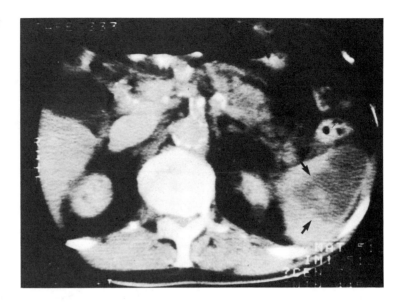

**Fig. 9-18.** *Major fracture of the midportion of the right kidney is evident (arrows). There is also extensive perirenal hematoma.*

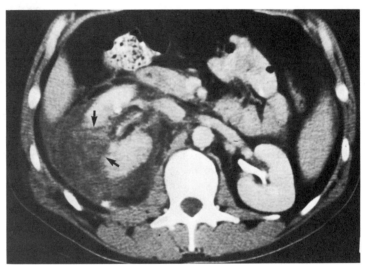

in these situations. Finally, it has the distinct advantage over other modalities in that head, thoracic, and abdominal information can be obtained during one examination.

E. **Xerography** is a process that is most applicable for depicting low-contrast objects with sharp, well-defined margins. It utilizes the charged surface of a photoconductor and forms an image after x-ray exposure; fine powder that is attracted to the conductor forms the visible image.

In the emergency setting, xerography is most useful in detecting **foreign bodies in the soft tissues.** It is more sen-

**Fig. 9-19.** *Multiple areas of traumatic contusion are present in the liver (arrows). The peritoneal lavage was negative, because the liver capsule was intact.*

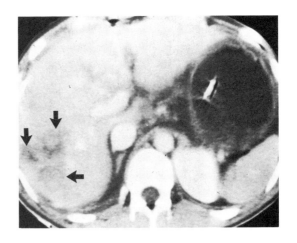

**Fig. 9-20.** *Percutaneous catheter drainage of a liver abscess.* **A.** *Large right lobe abscess in a patient with septicemia.* **B.** *After CT-guided catheter placement and evacuation of 350 ml of pus, the patient was cured.*

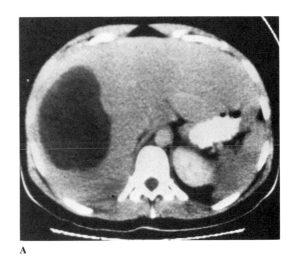

A

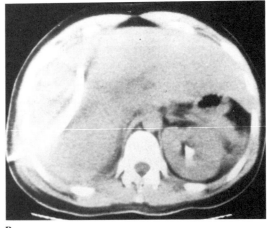

B

**Fig. 9-21.** *Percutaneous nephrostomy catheter relieves pyonephrosis caused by the staghorn calculus (arrow on filling defect in the renal pelvis, infundibulae, and calices).*

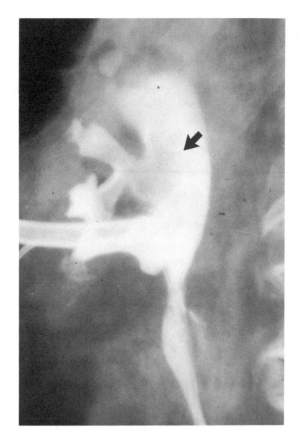

sitive than standard radiography for this purpose. The major uses are:

1. Suspected subcutaneous foreign bodies in wounds that are not seen on radiographs.
2. Localization and triangulation of superficial foreign bodies for surgical removal.
3. Diagnosis of ingested pharyngeal, laryngeal, or esophageal foreign bodies (e.g., chicken bone).

F. **Magnetic resonance imaging** (MRI) is a procedure whereby protons are excited by magnetization and the reactions are observed and recorded. Both images and spectroscopic information can be generated. Presently, MRI is most useful in the head and spinal cord. Imaging is comparable, or in some aspects, better than CT for certain thoracic and abdominal abnormalities. The practical application of these findings remains to be determined. MRI is not routine in emergency problems at present.

II. **Therapeutic interventional radiology in emergency situations.** Interventional radiology is a new field in radiology that is a coalescence of ultrasound, CT, and sophisticated needle and catheter techniques. It utilizes radiologic guidance (US, CT, fluo-

**Fig. 9-22.** *Emergency percutaneous biliary drainage temporizes septic, hypotensive elderly woman with jaundice. Catheter placed into the infected bile ducts permits decompression; note distal obstructing stone.*

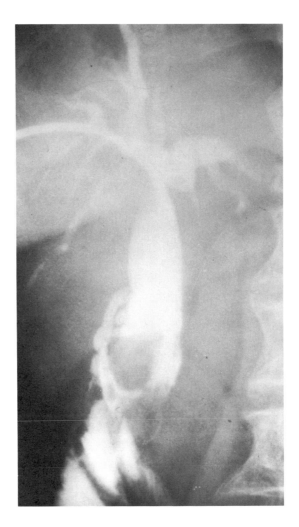

roscopy) to guide placement of instruments in the body and to treat the abnormalities that are detected by these imaging systems. Interventional radiology has important uses in the emergency room setting:

A. **Percutaneous abscess and fluid drainage.** This technique uses information from ultrasound and CT regarding location of abscesses and surrounding structures. This permits safe, guided insertion of a percutaneous catheter into the abscess. The cavity can be drained effectively in most abscesses (Fig. 9-20). Percutaneous abscess drainage is first-line treatment in most institutions.

B. **Percutaneous nephrostomy.** Catheters may be placed percutaneously to relieve obstructed kidneys. This technique usually is performed under fluoroscopy after opacification of the collecting system with contrast medium. The procedure also can be done directly with ultrasound guidance and without injection of intravenous contrast. Pyonephrosis may be drained by this method as well (Fig. 9-21).

**C. Percutaneous biliary drainage.** In a patient with cholangitis and sepsis due to biliary obstruction, percutaneous catheter decompression can relieve the acute problem and may be life-saving (Fig. 9-22). This usually will allow the patient's overall condition to improve prior to surgery. If there is incurable malignancy, the catheter may suffice for the duration of the patient's life. Percutaneous transhepatic cholangiography precedes this procedure.

**D. Angiographic control of gastrointestinal bleeding.** Once diagnostic angiography has determined a bleeding site, the catheter may be left in place to attempt control of the vessel. Pharmacologic agents or particles may be infused or injected through the catheter (see Fig. 9-14). This procedure has been particularly effective with bleeding gastritis.

SELECTED READINGS

Brant-Zawadzki M, Jeffrey RB Jr, Minagi H, et al. High resolution CT of thoracolumbar fractures. AJR 138:699, 1982.

Gelfand MJ. Scintigraphy in upper abdominal trauma. Semin Roentgenol 19:296, 1984.

Gomes MN. Clinical and surgical aspects of abdominal aortic aneurysms. SU 3:156, 1982.

Mueller PR, vanSonnenberg E, Ferrucci JT Jr. Percutaneous biliary drainage: Technical and catheter related problems in 200 procedures. AJR 138:17, 1982.

Schultz RD, Willi U. Sonography after blunt trauma in childhood. Radiology 152:255, 1984.

Shkolnik A. Applications of ultrasound in the neonatal abdomen. Radiol Clin North Am 23:141, 1985.

vanSonnenberg E, Casola G. Interventional Radiology—1988. Invest Radiol 23:75, 1988.

vanSonnenberg E, Mueller PR, Ferrucci JT Jr. Percutaneous drainage of 250 abdominal abscesses and fluid collections. Part I: Results, failures, and complications. Radiology 151:337, 1984.

# 10 The Recognition and Treatment of Contrast Reactions

*Eric vanSonnenberg and Richard C. Pfister*

Contrast reactions due to an intravenous urogram or a contrast-enhanced computed tomographic (CT) scan in the emergency setting generally is an unpredictable event. While those patients with prior reactions and atopic individuals are at greater risk (four and two times greater, respectively), the patient in whom a reaction will develop from any given examination cannot be identified beforehand. Skin testing has not proven effective and may induce a contrast reaction itself.

MECHANISMS

Reactions are divided into **mild, moderate,** and **severe.** The overall incidence of reactions is between 5 and 6 percent; most reactions are mild. Death is reported from 1 in 14,000 to 1 in 70,000. Contrast reactions are considered anaphylactoid, rather than truly allergic or anaphylactic for the following reasons: (1) prior contrast administration and therefore sensitization frequently has not occurred, (2) subsequent infusions of contrast medium do not necessarily induce similar (or any) reaction, and (3) incriminating antibodies to contrast or a haptene effect have not been demonstrated reliably. There is conflicting data with respect to antigen-antibody reactions and histamine release, such that true allergic mechanisms have not been documented.

A unified etiology for contrast reactions is undetermined, and it may be that there is an interplay of different mechanisms. These presumed mechanisms include anticholinesterase inhibition, activation of the complement system, antigen-antibody reaction, hyperosmolarity of the contrast medium, induction of histamine and other vasodilatory release mechanisms, cardiotoxic mechanisms, and even the psychological response.

Neither the type of contrast material that is used today (Hypaque, Conray, Renografin, Angiovist) nor the mode of infusion (drip or bolus) has been shown to make a significant difference in the incidence or severity of reactions (except bronchospasm with methylglucamine compounds). However, this area is one of con-

**Table 10-1.** *Management of Contrast Medium Reactions*

CLASS I REACTION TREATMENT

Nausea/vomiting

Check pulse and blood pressure, reassure the patient, discontinue injection then restart

Flushing, erythema

None

Hives, urticaria

1. Diphenhydramine (Benadryl) 50 mg IM or IV for itching
2. Observe: Be alert for insidious bronchospasm

Facial edema, conjunctivitis

1. Diphenhydramine (Benadryl) 50 mg IV
2. Rarely epinephrine 0.1 ml, 1 : 1000 SC
3. Observe: Be alert for insidious laryngeal edema

CLASS II REACTION TREATMENT

Bronchospasm, normotensive, normal heart

1. Oxygen by mask
2. Epinephrine 0.1−0.3 ml—1 : 1000 SC or 1 : 10,000 IV
3. Isoproterenol (Isuprel) aerosol inhalant
4. Possibly, Solu-Cortef 100 mg IV

Bronchospasm, normotensive, cardiac disease/elderly

1. Oxygen by mask
2. Aminophylline 500 mg in 50 ml D5W IV over 5−10 min

Bronchospasm, hypotensive

1. Normal heart: epinephrine 0.2−0.5 ml—1 : 1000 SC
   plus class III treatment
2. Cardiac disease/elderly: class III treatment

CLASS III REACTION TREATMENT

**Hypotension, vasodilative, normal heart, sinus rhythm**

1. Moderate with systolic blood pressure 60−80: **(a)** Trendelenburg position, **(b)** oxygen by mask, **(c)** baseline ECG, **(d)** emergency cart, **(e)** ask other personnel for assistance **(f)** start angiocath or intracath, **(g)** fluids IV rapidly over 30 min—1−2 liters normal saline or Ringer's lactate, **(h)** monitor pulse and blood pressure every 5 min and record
2. Severe with systolic blood pressure 40 or below or refractory, moderate hypotension/intolerance (cerebral, myocardial)
   **a.** Same as for moderate hypotension, steps **a** to **h,** plus vasopressor
   **b.** Insert CVP line and stethoscope lungs for CHF
       (1) High pressure: ephedrine 10−15 mg IV (may repeat in 15 min), or epinephrine 0.2−0.5 ml—1 : 1,000 SC
       (2) Low pressure: dopamine 200−400 $\mu$g/min titrated IV, or metaraminol (Aramine) 2−10 mg SC (may repeat in 10 min)
   **c.** Bicarbonate 44 mEq IV
   **d.** Solu-Cortef 100 mg IV

**Hypotension, vasodilative, cardiac disease/elderly, sinus rhythm,** moderate and severe: same as for normal heart, steps **a** to **f, (g)** CVP monitored (if CVP monitoring is not possible, auscultation of the lungs in hope of detecting pulmonary edema is essential), **(h)** 0.5−1.0 liter fluid cautiously, **(i)** dopamine 200 mg diluted and titrated 200−400 $\mu$g/min (epinephrine should be used cautiously or avoided), **(j)** Solu-Cortef 100 mg IV

**Hypotension (with or without vasodilation, heart disease), abnormal rate/rhythm (arrhythmia):** same as for normal heart, **a** to **f, (g)** CVP monitoring a necessity, **(h)** begin IV fluids, **(i)** Solu-Cortef 100 mg IV, **(j) sinus bradycardia:** atropine 1 mg IV; **A-V block and bradycardia:** isoproterenol (Isuprel) drip; **PVCs multifocal or 6/min unifocal:** lidocaine 100 mg IV; **ventricular tachycardia:** lidocaine bolus, then drip 1 mg/min; **asystole:** intracardiac epinephrine and CPR;

Table 10-1. (continued)

**electromechanical dissociation:** intracardiac epinephrine and CaCl$_2$; **ventricular fibrillation:** shock at 400 **watts-second** and CPR

OTHER DRUG TREATMENT

Convulsions: diazepam (Valium) 5 mg IV; total 10–20 mg prn; pento-barbital (Nembutal) 5 mg IV; total 100 mg prn; Note: Exclude hypotension as cause

Angina: nitroglycerin

Pulmonary edema: furosemide (Lasix) 20 mg IV

CVP = central venous pressure; CHF = congestive heart failure; A-V = atrioventricular; PVC = premature ventricular contraction; CPR = cardiopulmonary resuscitation.

tinued investigation at present. Direct injection into a central line is inadvisable, as this may be arrhythmogenic. The newer nonionic agents do appear to have fewer reactions. As such, they are recommended for patients who have had prior reactions. Steroid pretreatment has been proven to be effective in countering reactions due to the ionic contrast media. The preferred dosage is sequential methyl prednisone tablets the day before and the day of the examination.

Reactions usually occur immediately after the infusion has begun. Most reactions are manifested within 5 minutes; occasionally, however, they will not develop for 15 to 20 minutes.

Close observation of patients who are intubated, comatose, or with marginally maintained blood pressure is mandatory in the emergency setting; the patient unexpectedly may become severely hypotensive, due either to vasodilatory effects of contrast or to a cardiogenic effect (ectopy, arrhythmia, bradycardia, ischemia). Routine monitoring of the heart during intravenous urography (IVU) has shown both ST–T changes and conduction abnormalities.

TREATMENT

**Mild reactions** (class I) generally require no treatment or treatment of symptoms at most (Table 10-1). The symptoms include a feeling of flush or heat, nausea and vomiting, tingling in the extremities, and perioral numbness. These usually are transient and, with physician assurance, as a rule are self-limited. Mild cutaneous symptoms and signs including erythema and itching may be treated with diphenhydramine (Benadryl) 25 or 50 mg orally or intramuscularly. Local extravasation of contrast in a vein can be treated with elevation and heat.

**Moderate reactions** include the following:

1. **Wheezing,** due to bronchospasm rather than pulmonary edema. Pulmonary edema is an extremely rare complication of contrast reactions.
2. More marked **cutaneous manifestations.**
3. **Lightheadedness,** which can be due to a vasovagal effect with bradycardia.

**10. The Recognition and Treatment of Contrast Reactions** **301**

**Bronchospasm** (class II) is treated with subcutaneous **epinephrine** 1/1000, 0.3 ml, which may be repeated (or IV 1/10,000 0.1–0.3 ml) **oxygen** and, if necessary, **aminophylline** 500 mg in 50 ml of D5W over 15 minutes (see Table 10-1). The more marked cutaneous manifestations can be treated with 0.3 ml of epinephrine subcutaneously. Patients with moderate reactions must be observed carefully for about an hour to be certain that their clinical condition does not deteriorate. Vasovagal bradycardia is treated with 0.6 to 1.2 mg IV atropine.

The **most severe** reaction is **hypotension** (class III), and this can be moderate or severe and life-threatening (see Table 10-1). Symptoms that may herald the hypotension are lightheadedness, dyspnea, syncope, chills, nausea and vomiting, and chest pain. Seizures or severe cutaneous manifestations also may be the mode of presentation; however, cutaneous signs and symptoms are not present invariably. Probable mechanisms of hypotension include vasovagal attacks and/or liberation of vasodilators including histamine. A cardiogenic etiology also must be ruled out (myocardial infarction or ischemia, arrhythmia) as a cause of major hypotension and shock.

Dyspnea with stridor from **laryngeal edema** is another manifestation of a **severe** reaction. Epinephrine (1/1000 0.3 ml subsequently or 1/10,000 5 ml IV), steroids IV (e.g., Solucortef 100 mg IV) are administered. Endotracheal or cricothyroid intubation may be required.

It is the patient who is obtunded or for some reason cannot communicate in whom the hypotensive reaction may go unnoticed. Therefore, frequent monitoring of these patients in the emergency setting is mandatory. It is important to emphasize the adage that **no critically injured or ill patient should be unattended in the radiology department.**

The mechanism of severe hypotension in contrast reactions probably is marked reduction in peripheral vascular resistance due to vasodilatation, and therefore effective hypovolemia. Hypovolemic, dehydrated patients should be replenished as well as possible **prior** to administration of contrast.

**Treatment of major reactions**

1. Initial evaluation of the cardiovascular and pulmonary status of the patient is done. Blood pressure and pulse determination and auscultation of the heart and lungs are performed.
2. **Contrast** infusion is **stopped** immediately. Contrast is flushed out of the tubing with normal saline.
3. The patient is placed in the **Trendelenburg position** and the legs are elevated on pillows for immediate autotransfusion.
4. **Fluids** should be infused rapidly via the initial line for the contrast infusion and with a second **large-bore catheter** (central

**Fig. 10-1.** *Hypotensive nephrogram. After intravenous contrast administration, there is no excretion of contrast in the collecting systems of the kidneys. The kidneys continued to become dense and eventually shrank in length due to poor perfusion associated with the patient's hypotension.*

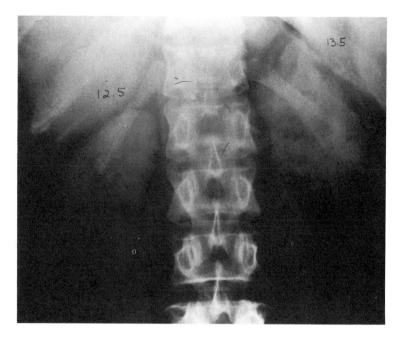

if possible). One-half to two liters of normal saline and occasionally albumin may be necessary to restore the blood pressure. Frequent auscultation and central venous pressure monitoring are done to be certain pulmonary edema does not develop. **Volume replacement has proven to be an effective and safe method to treat contrast-induced hypotension** (as in other forms of effective hypovolemic shock).

5. **Oxygen** is administered. Flow is limited to 2 to 4 liters/min in patients with chronic obstructive pulmonary disease (COPD).
6. **ECG** is performed.
   a. For **sinus bradycardia, atropine** should be administered intravenously in 0.6 to 1.2 mg dosage.
   b. For **significant ventricular ectopy, lidocaine** bolus (75 mg) and a drip (2 mg/min) may be necessary.
7. The **airway** must be **cleared** of secretions by suctioning.
8. **Steroids** have not been proven to be beneficial, but can be administered in high doses intravenously (Solucortef 100 mg) without harm.
9. **Seizures** are best managed by **treating the hypotension** and hypoxemia as above. Occasionally diazepam or pentobarbital IV may be needed.
10. **Drugs.** Epinephrine (intravenously 1/10,000 in a dose of 0.5 ml, or 0.5 ml in a 1:1,000 drip in 10 ml of sodium chloride) has been a standard agent for treatment of major reactions. However, prudence with sympathomimetic drugs is important in patients with underlying COPD and hypoxemia or underlying

ischemic heart disease, lest severe arrhythmias be induced. In the patient with hypotension and a new arrhythmia, those drugs with arrhythmogenic properties may be more deleterious than beneficial. Aramine, norepinephrine, and phenylephrine also must be used with caution. **Dopamine** is particularly valuable to improve inotropism when volume has been restored. **Antihistamines** are not advocated in the acute hypotensive setting.

The major late complication of a contrast reaction is acute renal failure. This can be particularly severe in the patient who is hypovolemic prior to the study and becomes hypotensive with resultant acute tubular necrosis. Hypovolemia must be avoided, particularly in the traumatized patient. Diabetic patients and those in renal failure, and patients with multiple myeloma are at particular risk.

In a **hypotensive reaction,** the IVU initially will demonstrate a **poor nephrogram** effect and minimal to no contrast in the collecting systems bilaterally. This is due to **diminished renal perfusion** and not necessarily renal disease per se. In time the nephrogram intensifies, but excretion is poor. The renal size may decrease, due to impaired blood flow into the kidney (Fig. 10-1).

SELECTED READINGS

Andrews EJ Jr. Vagus reaction as a possible cause of severe complications of radiological procedures. Radiology 121:1, 1976.

Bagg MNJ, Horwitz TA, Bester L. Comparison of patient responses to high- and low-osmolality contrast agents injected intravenously. AJR 147:185, 1986.

Dawson P. Contrast agent nephrotoxicity. An appraisal. Radiology 157:568, 1985.

Lasser EC, Berry CC, Talner LB, et al. Pretreatment with corticosteroids to alleviate reactions to intravenous contrast material. N Engl J Med 317:845, 1987.

Loughran CF. Clinical intravenous urography: Comparative trial of ioxaglate and iopamidol. Radiology 161:455, 1986.

Pfister RC, Hutter AM Jr. Cardiac alterations during intravenous urography. Invest Radiol 15:S239, 1980.

Scott WR. Seizures: A reaction to contrast media for computed tomography of the brain. Radiology 137:359, 1980.

Shehadi WH, Toniolo G. Adverse reactions to contrast media: A report from the Committee on Safety of Contrast Media of the International Society of Radiology. Radiology 137:299, 1980.

Spring DB, Akin Jr, Margulis AR. Informed consent for intravenous contrast-enhanced radiography: A national survey of practice and opinion. Radiology 152:609, 1984.

Thomas ML, Keeling FP, Piaggio RB, et al. Contrast agent induced thrombophlebitis following leg phlebography: Iopamidol versus meglumine iothalamate. Radiology 153:564, 1984.

vanSonnenberg E, Neff CC, Pfister RC. Life-threatening hypotensive reactions to contrast media administration: Comparison of pharmacologic and fluid therapy. Radiology 162:15, 1987.

# 11 Guidelines for X-ray Studies During Pregnancy

*Eric vanSonnenberg and Michael P. André*

The marked radiosensitivity of the early embryo and developing fetus dictates great care in avoidance of unnecessary radiography during pregnancy. Complications to the fetus from exposure to radiation include death (the very early embryo, especially preimplantation stage), congenital malformations (the nervous system being most readily damaged), and possibly malignancy (increased leukemia susceptibility).

The problem in making specific recommendations to a mother who has been radiated is that knowledge of radiation effects in the fetus are based largely on experimental evidence in mice and rats (which may or may not be extrapolated to humans) and on the effects of large radiation doses to humans that occurred at Hiroshima and Nagasaki. Precise dosages that cause damage are not agreed on by all authors. Generally, below a 10-rad dose (rad = unit of absorbed radiation dose), concern about damage is speculative. Exposure between 10 to 25 rads causes cellular changes. More than 25 rads may induce malformations and growth retardation. The fetus in its first trimester undergoes organogenesis, and hence is most susceptible to malformations in this period. The risk of leukemia from low-dose radiation is controversial (some studies have found a correlation, others have not).

The preceding must be integrated with the specific indication for the x-ray. If the indication is nonelective and crucial in the care of the mother (and hence the fetus), the x-ray should be performed according to the consensus of the American College of Radiology and the National Council on Radiation Protection. Abdominal and pelvic procedures (barium enema, intravenous urography, hip and lumbar spine series, upper gastrointestinal series) have the highest dosage to the uterus (Table 11-1). The maximum permissible dose to the fetus from occupational exposure of the mother is 0.5 rem per year.

Difficulty in determining the need for radiography arises when

**Table 11-1.** *Estimated Average Embryonic or Fetal Dose per Diagnostic Radiologic Examination*

| Examination | Dose to embryo (millirads) |
|---|---|
| Skull | 4 |
| Cervical spine | 2 |
| Upper extremity | 1 |
| Lower extremity | 1 |
| Shoulder | 1 |
| Chest | |
|    Radiography | 8 |
|    Fluoroscopy | 70 |
| Thoracic spine | 9 |
| Upper gastrointestinal series | |
|    Radiography | 360 |
|    Fluoroscopy | 200 |
|    Total | 560 |
| Barium enema | |
|    Radiography | 440 |
|    Fluoroscopy | 360 |
|    Total | 800 |
| Cholecystography | 200 |
| Intravenous or retrograde pyelography | 400 |
| Abdomen | 290 |
| Lumbar spine | 275 |
| Pelvis | 40 |
| Hip | 300 |
| Ultrasound | 0 |
| Magnetic resonance imaging | 0 |
| Computed tomography | 2000* |

*If in the field of exposure. The fetal dose decreases by a factor of three every two inches that the fetus is from the nearest computed tomographic section (e.g., if two inches distant, fetal dose would be 667 millirads; if four inches distant, 222 millirads).

symptoms of pregnancy mistakenly suggest abdominal disease (cramping, nausea, vomiting). Another problem is that in the first few weeks after conception, when the embryo is **most** vulnerable, the urinary pregnancy test may be negative. This has prompted the so-called 10-day rule. It states that "radiation of women of child-bearing age should be restricted to within 10 days after onset of menstruation." Thus the chance of harming the fetus in an unsuspected early pregnancy is virtually excluded. However, this might have genetic implications, since a certain percentage of women would then have had radiation (ovaries included) just prior to conception, thereby creating a pool of affected ova that subsequently could be impregnated. Both these hypotheses are somewhat speculative, and, fortunately, deal with a very small segment of women in the reproductive years. Therefore, the specific need for the x-ray should take precedence.

Another source of confusion that may influence decisions is an ectopic pregnancy, in which there is abdominal pain and tenderness and the pregnancy test may be positive. Ultrasonography is the procedure of choice and frequently will clarify the problem.

Guidelines and recommendations for x-rays during pregnancy include the following (adapted from the National Council on Radiation Protection and Measurements):

1. Nonessential and elective radiation should be avoided.
2. The care of an immediate problem is paramount for the mother (and subsequently for the fetus); therefore, indicated studies should be performed.
3. Radiation should be limited by filtration, collimation, shielding of the mother and fetus, and avoidance of low-yield views.
4. If there has been abdominal or pelvic radiation in the first half of the menstrual cycle, conception might best be delayed for 1 to 2 months.
5. A heavy exposure (greater than 10 rads) probably requires consultation regarding pregnancy interruption.
6. Less risky (i.e., lack of harmful radiation) diagnostic studies should be substituted when possible during pregnancy. Ultrasound and magnetic resonance imaging may be preferable in these cases.

SELECTED READINGS

Bhatnagar JP, Gorson RO, Krohmer JS. X-ray doses to patients undergoing full-spine radiographic examination. Radiology 138:231, 1981.

Faulkner K, Gordon MDH, Miller J. Detailed study of radiation dose and radiographic technique during chest radiography. Br J Radiol 59:245, 1986.

Gustafsson M, Mortensson W. Radiation exposure and estimate of late effects of chest roentgen examination in children. Acta Radiol (Diagn) 24 (Fasc. 4):309, 1983.

Moilanen A, Kokko M-L, Pitkanen M. Gonadal dose reduction in lumbar spine radiography. Radiology 1499:153, 1983.

National Council on Radiation Protection and Measurements. Review of NCRP Radiation Dose Limit for Embryo and Fetus in Occupationally Exposed Women, NCRP Report 53, 1977.

National Council on Radiation Protection and Measurements. Medical Radiation Exposure of Pregnant and Potentially Pregnant Women, NCRP Report 54, 1977.

Ragozzino MW, Gray JE, Burke TM, Van Lysel MS. Estimation and minimalization of fetal absorbed dose: Data from common radiographic examinations. AJR 137:667, 1981.

Sabau MN, Radkowski MA, Vyborny CJ. Radiation exposure due to scatter in neonatal radiographic procedures. AJR 144:811, 1985.

Webster EW. On the question of cancer introduction by small x-ray doses. AJR 137:647, 1981.

Wood JW, Johnson KG, Omori Y. In utero exposure to the Hiroshima atomic bomb: An evaluation of head size and mental retardation: Twenty years later. Pediatrics 39 (3), 1967.

# Index

Italic page numbers refer to figures; page numbers followed by "*t*" refer to tables.